SELF DEFENSE

Easy and Effective Self Protection Whatever Your Age

(The Ultimate Guide to Beginner Martial Arts Training Techniques)

Jason Bernard

Published by Phil Dawson

Jason Bernard

All Rights Reserved

Self Defense: Easy and Effective Self Protection Whatever Your Age (The Ultimate Guide to Beginner Martial Arts Training Techniques)

ISBN 978-1-77485-304-7

Legal & Disclaimer

The information contained in this book is not designed to replace or take the place of any form of medicine or professional medical advice. The information in this book has been provided for educational and entertainment purposes only.

The information contained in this book has been compiled from sources deemed reliable, and it is accurate to the best of the Author's knowledge; however, the Author cannot guarantee its accuracy and validity and cannot be held liable for any errors or omissions. Changes are periodically made to this book. You must consult your doctor or get professional medical advice before using any of the suggested remedies, techniques, or information in this book.

TABLE OF CONTENTS

Introduction

This book provides a reference to understand US gun laws, the rights to own guns and when it is legal permissible to carry a gun.

It is a controversial topic in light of a number of incident of shootings that been in the news. There are a variety of issues that have been raised, including:

When is it safe to carry guns?

Is it legal to fire an employee?

Since these are sensitive topics all responsible citizens and especially gun owners must be familiar with the basic principles about these rules.

Learn more.

Chapter 1: Pressure Point Fighting? No Pressure

If you ask a hundred martial practitioners regarding pressure points, and ways to make use of them in self-defense and you'll get around hundred of different responses. Pressure point combat is a traditional fighting method or art form, or whatever you want to refer to it as.

It's actually referred to by numerous names. In Japan they refer to it as Kyusho Jitsu. On other hand, some refer to it Ryukyu Kempo. In China they refer to it Dim Mak. If you're looking to sound serious and humorous while still sounding serious it is possible to describe it as the death touch or simply the death point striking.

That last line does make this sound as if it's a film however, there was actually a film with the same title.

The most important thing to remember is that the definition of pressure point combat will be determined by the person who you are asking. It all is dependent on the system of martial arts or the background that the other person comes from.

Some might dismiss it as just a myth. Some might exaggerate and make it seem absurd. There are also people who actually apply it, and can give you a useful lesson - something you can apply for self-defense.

The Myth of the Myth

One of the myths you've heard of is that of a martial arts master who was able to take down or knock down his adversaries with just a flick the tip of his hand. That sounds something like Kung Fu Panda with Po doing the Skadoosh move using his pinky finger.

The original story isn't as vibrant or hilarious as the others. In certain versions of the legend, it spoke of certain Kung fu masters that were able to defeat their adversaries using simple techniques that weren't deadly. In some versions , the masters of kungfu were shown to being zen masters that could kill a person at the stroke of the finger.

It is possible to say that the story itself sparked a lot of imaginative thinking. Apart from Po the other character that immediately comes to mind - Spock. Spock. Do you remember Spock's Vulcan nerve pinch? Well people refer to it as"the Vulcan grip. Just one touch to the neck's back regardless of whether you're human or not you'll be out for the count.

A different movie-inspired method of fighting with pressure points is one of the techniques explained by The Kill Bill movies: the five-point palm explosion heart technique. Just one touch and you're just five steps. The next thing you'll notice is the moment that you feel your heart go off within your chest, and you collapse to the ground in a dead state. That's the way it is according to the film made by Quentin Tarantino.

These facts are allusions to the legend's origins. We are given the following details from the legend and mythology of The death touch

The pressure points can be involved

The strikes may not appear deadly, but they are

You need to be skilled expert to perform it

Certain effects may be delayed

The last sentence there was speculation that what killed the legend Bruce Lee was a death punch or death touch (whatever you prefer to label it). Maybe he was a practicing one of his friends and the death touch was sprayed (intentionally or accidentally). Naturally, the degeneration of Lee's organs did not occur in a hurry.

The incident occurred a few hours later and caused Bruce Lee's death. Then, as per the theory of this, Bruce Lee died of the death contact. Unfortunately, we won't learn.

What is the Truth Behind the Myth

Are you curious to know where "death touch" originated? It's not necessary to search far for the name was popularized because of a number of commercials that were aired during the 60s and 70s.

In the past, full-page ads were published for Marvel comics. The ad featured a character named Count Dante. Naturally, the advertisement was promoting a book, an martial arts book. What was the title of"the art of fighting? Yes, it's the Death Touch as taught by the Count Dante as well as his so-called Black Dragon Society.

Commotio Cordis

Before you dismiss the idea off, you should consider this medically-proven and scientifically researched phenomenon known as Commotio Cordis. It's a fatality resulted by a blow to the chest area of a person that disrupts the heart rhythm.

You can't kill the heart, and it isn't exploding. Actually the heart is still functioning. However, the electrical signals which control heartbeat are disrupted, as is the heart's rhythm.

The disturbance to the heart's rhythm is enough to cause death. The chest strike will occur in a small time frame - around 10 to 30 milliseconds, to be precise.

Does this really happen? Is it true?

The answer is yes.

In actual fact there are more than 100 documented cases of Commotio cordis. Certain cases involve hockey players who were hit by a hockey ball in the exact spot and precisely at the right moment.

Don't be scared to hit someone accidentally with your chest. You have a one out of a million chances of causing commotion chordis. you need to be exact and robust to be able to do it.

So, what exactly is Pressure Point Combating Really?

To simplify things Pressure point fighting, as well as self-defense makes the use of pressure points during combat situations. A pressure point is area of the body where nerve endings are close to the skin , in such a way that applying pressure enough will trigger a reaction in the body.

Certain pressure points can be used to treat. However some pressure points may be utilized to create dizziness, pain as well as other side effects including knocking the other person out. It's not knockouts as in boxing terms however, it could be.

Pressure can be applied to these pressure points by various methods. One method is to massage these points. There are a variety of pressure point treatments that help ease the pain, enhance body functions, and aid in treating various ailments.

But striking certain pressure points with your fists, hands or knees, elbows, and kicks can result in injury (which is exactly what you'd like to avoid doing if you're seeking to protect yourself).

What is the impact on the body when a key pressure point on the body is hit in order to fight? Here are a few consequences:

Confusion loss

Balance is disturbed

Extreme pain

A stunning effect

Motor dysfunction

There are, of course, pressure points and strategies you can use to knock someone else out. knocking someone out isn't always a way of knocking out the person like you would when you box with punches.

According to the martial art in practiced, knocking out can mean a variety of things. For instance, according to some martial arts practitioners who practice karate, hitting the "knockout tension point" could result in dizziness. For them, it's already thought of as a knockout.

To make it easier for you to comprehend To make things easier to comprehend, a knockout can be the point at which your opponent is in a position to be in a position to not attack you. It could happen when they are briefly stunned, permitting you to flee. It could be that you've stopped your opponent from moving or after you have armed your opponent and are now in control of the situation.

In any confrontation where you've achieved a decisive advantage (and the health or life of the opponent is in your own hands and, in the best case scenario,) If you have a decisive advantage, then you should think of it as knockout. It's important to remember that knockouts are not always a boxer's idea.

Knockout Pressure Points

This could be the haymaker's question Is there a pressure point one can touch, press or strike to knock out the other person or end his life? The idea is a bit nebulous.

It is true that knockout pressure points can be a bit vague. In the realistic sense of street combat where everything is unpredictable the only reasonable definition of a knockout would be when the opponent has lost their consciousness.

There are two kinds of pressure points that could create this kind of impact:

Pressure points that limit the blood flow - the rear naked choke, for example.

Impact pressure points are similar to an ax on the jaw.

Since we're already on the topic, there are three distinct methods or styles for pressure point combat:

Impact-related (punches, knees and kicks and other methods of striking)

Limitation of blood flow

The pain-inducing

In the next section, we'll discuss the various goals you should strive at. But, there's a piece of advice that is of practical is to be aware that no amount of reading can beat hours of practicing at the gym.

You can study the fundamentals by reading this book, however, if you desire to master the art of protect yourself from harm, then you must to find a real instructor who can train you. Also, you need someone who will train you (that must be one who is willing to experience the pain from every single pressure point you'll hit).

Your trainer will assist you in learning to handle the hurt (of course, you'll get struck too).

Be realistic about your expectations. Don't assume that because you are familiar with self-defense techniques that you'll come through a fight without injury. No sir. If you get involved in an argument, you'll be hurt the majority times.

A practical tip prevention remains the most effective defense for yourself that is available. If you are able to keep a cool head and avoid situations where you could be injured, then you've successfully applied the best self defense techniques available.

Chapter 2: Self-Defense Basics

It's an easy method that can provide you with an excellent foundation upon which you can construct. Finding out how to avoid the threat is important aspect of self-defense when you're just beginning your learning. This book will provide the basics and basic concepts you can to apply to a variety of scenarios. You might want to further train.

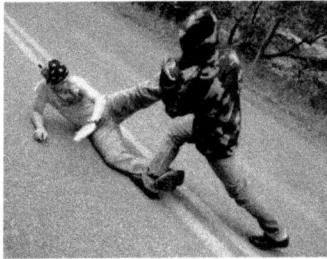

The Basics

Make a plan of attack to avoid danger. Avoidance is the first priority, but when this fails you, then the next step should be escape. Avoidance is dependent on your awareness, which can be increased by enhancing your self-defense skills by studying and reading.

If walking or running away isn't your option, the escape route is your next option. If it's an actual fight, you must try to make the encounter as brief as is possible. If you let it drag on the odds are against you.

If you're in the process of learning not to get caught up in an urgency to get through and learn the next techniques. Be patient and allow the concepts sink in.

It is a collection of various concepts. It's more simple to grasp a couple of concepts rather than learning the exact method to defend against any kind of attack.

We've adopted several of the fundamental concepts that are used to create various breaks and breakaway techniques, paired with some basic hitting and placement. Together, they'll give you good understanding basic self-defense techniques.

You may currently live in an area that you believe is secure and not necessary for this type of novel, but do you think it will remain as it is now? Are you seeing the region grow by bringing new people in with different ideas and values them? Are you planning to leave the region to go on a trip to work or for to have fun? It may be useful just to get some fresh ideas. Be open to new ideas and take an examination of the situation in a different way It's not a bad idea being prepared for what could happen.

These methods utilize gross motor skills (basic body motions) which makes them incredibly simple to master and apply. The techniques or concepts must be simple to use under stress.

These are crucial factors since methods must be simple enough to be executed under stress. Practice these strategies with your friends and family members. The more practice you do, the more natural they'll feel.

Also, practice your newly learned abilities in various places, such as in the kitchen, bathroom and front room, garage, and so on. If you are spending a lot or all of the time within smaller spaces or rooms, do not limit your training to the vast gymnasium's open area. You must train in environments that are suitable to your needs.

To increase your awareness, it's helpful to know who the enemy is and be able to discern their actions, and even the practices that are common to different kinds of attackers. Women are more likely to meet a different type of attacker that men will be expected to confront. Women are more likely to attack men as muggers and rapists, in contrast to males.

If we can understand the adversary and understand the enemy, we stand the best likelihood of winning the battle of them. There's a lot of deceit that goes with these types of people, and generally the more serious the crime, the greater the chance of deceit. There are many people who match the stereotype of "The The Bad Guy" and often you won't have to look past your own close ones. We hear stories of violence in the home on a daily day basis.

Be careful not to be caught in your personal bubble and keep in mind that there are other people who are not in your area. It doesn't matter whether we like it or not, there are some people who's goals don't always work out for the best. Maybe you'll never meet those who behave like this, but there is a chance that you might or maybe you have already encountered. It could be at your workplace, at home or on the street at a bar or even in the street It could be anywhere. Don't be afraid to turn off the lights, because that's exactly the kind of person that vultures hunt.

Sometimes, bad things occur to the best of people, so don't believe that it can't happen to you since it may. I'm not saying it won't happen, but it could. There are reports of things occurring all the time and just knowing that there's a problem is a major step.

Chapter 3: State Laws On Guns And Self-Defense

The question of whether it appropriate and legal to carry guns is not simple. The legality of use is contingent on a variety of factors and the opinion of the judge and/or the jury. Additionally, the law enforcement personnel who arrive on the site will also have distinct opinions about the issue.

State Laws regarding Civil Lawsuits

Because there are numerous opinions and various elements in playing in determining what's legally acceptable, states have various laws that govern this matter. Some state legislatures have passed legislation to shield individuals from civil court proceedings that are filed by families of criminals. Certain states do not offer this protection, and allow families of the criminal (or their families of attackers) to bring civil lawsuits regarding the using deadly force against relatives of the attackers. In certain states, even though the use of deadly force in self-defense has been previously justified.

State Laws regarding "Third Parties"

Additionally, many States have legislation that permit an individual to use deadly force to protect self or other innocent persons. Certain states have specified "third parties" as innocents who are at risk that have caused a person to resort to deadly force to defend those in danger.

In Oklahoma innocents or third parties who could justify the need to use force to defend themselves include the following individuals:

Parent

Husband

Widow

Child/children

Mistress

Master

Servant

In Vermont the list is used for innocents or other third parties who are who are in danger, which can justify the usage of force to kill and includes the following additions:

The wife

Husband

Child

Parent

Sister

Brother

Guardian

Ward

Mistress

Master

Servant

Laws of the State Laws in relation to Ability to Retrench

Refraining is an essential element in the legal reasoning behind the lethal force used. States have differing opinions on this matter. Certain states have laws that oblige the first step is to flee when confronted by an attacker. Use of deadly force only occurs when there is no option. If someone has had a an opportunity to escape or escape from the situation, but decided to resort to the force of death, he or she could be charged with murder.

States with laws that provide for obligation to withdraw if the attack occurs in the home. These include:

Arkansas

Alaska

Connecticut

District of Columbia

Delaware

Hawaii

Maine

Iowa

Maryland

New Hampshire

Minnesota

New Jersey

New York

South Carolina

Nebraska

North Dakota

Ohio

Rhode Island

Pennsylvania

Wyoming

Castle Doctrine

The majority of states have adopted this policy. It states that individuals are not under any obligation to withdraw when faced by a life-threatening threat, whether it occurs at workplace or at home.

The doctrine of this kind is based on an ancient and well-established principle of law that states that the home of a person can be described as a castle. The owner of the castle has the instinctual desire to defend their castle at all costs including using violent force when the situation requires it. Any resident of that castle has the legal right to defend the castle.

Although the doctrine is founded on a standard legal principle, the way it is applied differs from state the state. In certain states the law is applicable to both threats to individuals as well as property. In other states the doctrine is restricted to threats only to individuals. In addition, the term "home" is defined in different ways in the various states. Certain states define "home" as just the home. Certain states extend this definition to work and business locations or even one's own automobile.

The doctrine, though it may be a good concept, could be dangerous in certain instances. In particular, this idea has led to the loss of lives, many that ended in death as a result of entering a house in error. For example, a mentally impaired person who was confused, drunk or under the influence of drugs entered the home of someone else accidentally and was confronted by a deadly force.

To stay clear of these unlucky circumstances to prevent this from happening, the statute on the ability to withdraw is incorporated into the laws of certain states.

State Laws on the Use of deadly force

There aren't many states with laws that specify the use of force in self-defense. Certain states have laws but others have unclear laws. Certain states have no laws whatsoever and simply adapt the court case law as a the basis for jury instructions and cases. They include:

Illinois

California

Rhode Island

Ohio

District of Columbia

New Mexico

Idaho

West Virginia

Massachusetts

Maryland

North Carolina

South Carolina

New Mexico

Oklahoma

Some states have an open approach regarding the justification for "use of force that is deadly". One of these states is Texas. The law in Texas permits the use of force against a individual if the one who used force was able to demonstrate good reason to believe it was necessary due to imminent or immediate danger of death or serious bodily injury.

The definitions of "imminent" and "immediate" is different for states. Furthermore, some states will require justifiable grounds beyond "imminent as well as urgent" dangers. States that are like these:

Maryland

North Carolina

District of Columbia

California

Rhode Island

North Dakota

Idaho

Colorado

Massachusetts

The states also require individuals to make use of minimal force to defend oneself. This means that using deadly force could not be justified if, on reviewing, there were other methods to defend oneself.

States such as South Carolina and New Mexico have more to say on this specific point. The use of deadly force is also justified in the event that a person with the same courage and determination would have followed the same path or believed the same when confronted with the same circumstance.

The State's Laws regarding "Stand Your Ground"

"Stand your ground" or the "stand on your feet" concept is an expansion of Castle doctrine. This implies that citizens are allowed to use force confronted with danger, even in the presence of strangers.

The state laws permits a person to remain in place and defend them and the property they own (i.e. homes, residences as well as their place of business or work, etc.) against any imminent or apparent threat. There is no obligation to withdraw if the person is entitled to remain there at the moment. Also, there is a legal right to apply any form of force, including the use of deadly force, if there is a good reason to believe that a threat to serious physical or bodily harm is immediate and imminent.

The law is heavily influenced by it's Castle doctrine, wherein certain state laws have expanded beyond the mere place of residence to areas that a person is entitled to be during a specific moment.

One instance is one example is the "stand your feet" laws in Michigan. It stipulates that individuals do not have the obligation to withdraw from a spot in which he is legally entitled to be. It is so in the event that the person is honest and has reasonable reason to think that using force will protect him from serious physical injury or death. Michigan law permits this to the use of deadly force to prevent sexual assault the person who is assaulted or on someone else.

Some states have adopted the same law. Some examples include Georgia and Indiana which have recently enacted this law amid worries that existing laws might be replaced by the concept of "duty to withdraw". California, Virginia and a handful of other states have enacted the law, but there aren't any laws in place. The law in West Virginia, this law has been in place for some time, however it the law was codified only in the year 2008.

Colorado has a different version of the law, known as "no obligation to retreat". It is based on the same concept but applies to people who were the aggressors in the first place. For example, individuals who might have caused the conflict are initially required to "retreat to the wall" or attempt to get out of the situation. If retreat does not stop the threat's escalation The aggressor might have a legitimate reason to resort to using force to resolve the threat or conflict.

Chapter 4: The 3 A's - Awareness, Assessment, and Assertiveness

The first step towards self-defense is to be aware. Recognize what your weaknesses and strengths are, know your strengths and weaknesses. You must be aware of your weaknesses and identify any attacks and plan your options prior to the time.

If you're employed in an establishment that requires you to work late at night on your own, you must know the weaknesses of your job. Think about what could be the worst thing that could happen to me while I'm working my shift at your cash counter? What might happen when I close the shop and locking the shop from to the street?

Being aware also means that you are mindful and alert all the time to avoid an incident that could be violent. The age-old saying "An an ounce of prevention is better than a pound cure" is equally applicable for us. Criminals are always looking for weak and unwary prey. It's a good idea to portray a picture that tells people to be cautious and you are serious about business. Keep your head elevated and keep watching people who are passing on the other side or walking in front of you. Attackers typically target their victims at the time they are least expecting that, which is why it's always advantageous to be aware of an attack.

Wear clothes that make it easier to defend yourself and not give other people weaknesses to attack. When you get home, put on shoes from your office shoes to help you move more easily. Choose a bag to help you keep your arms free. For example, a bag that has an extended strap that you can carry over your shoulder or backpack. If you have hair that is long put it in the shape of a bun or put it inside your coat so that no one can get the hair. The ponytail isn't ideal since someone could tug at it. Therefore, avoid wearing necklaces or scarves that can be used to strangle. Also, wearing extravagant jewelry could make you a victim. In addition, you should avoid having one of the senses shut off. Wear contacts or glasses for those who have problems with vision and avoid using an MP3 player which could cause you to be deaf to the the world. Remove your mobile device or tablet that could be distracting and could also draw the attention of muggers.

Be aware of the surroundings. While walking back to your car, determine the most efficient route with enough lighting and room to run in case of need. It is even better to ask for a companion to walk alongside you.

Do a thorough evaluation of your circumstances and potential solutions you have available to you. Utilize the resources you have to make the most of the adversity. If you are working all night in a retail store maybe it's wise to request the store's manager to set up security measures at the shop particularly if you're situated in a particularly dangerous neighborhood. Security cameras, alarms, and a door that has locks that are safe are great not only for you, but also for the shop. It is also possible to keep an item like a bat on the counter or request the counter to be protected by a bulletproof glass window to be put in. You should have a door and grate that is easy to lock or close when you leave. It can be a long time trying to get the grates back and using keys on padlocks that weigh a lot will give attackers enough time to plot their assault against you.

Additionally, consider your physical condition. Did you have a track star in high school and a fast-paced runner with strong legs that can give an amazing kick? Do you have nails that are long which you could use to scratch at attackers? Are you small, and could be able to get through the cracks in the side of the street? Be aware of your body, and the things that it has against the big muscled criminal.

If the argument is occurring, make sure you are confident. It is still possible to stop a physical assault by speaking and trying to figure out what the other person's needs.

If it's just cash or your mobile phone and you are not sure, it's ideal to leave it and let the criminal leave, particularly in the event that you've determined that you're in a disadvantage. The mugger might be firing a gun towards you or being surrounded by multiple attacker. Be mindful of your safety first. take action when you're already in a safe place by contacting the police and providing all the information you know about the person who attacked you.

However, if the conflict is already physical and physical, then make lots of noise and then start trying to fight back. If the criminal didn't expect you to take on the challenge, it is enough to deter him from pursuing the fight. It is not the right moment to dress up and appear sexy. Make sure you assert your authority on your own body, space and your possessions that no one can ever take your possessions.

Chapter 5: Security At Work For Women

It's quite a shock when you discover that women aren't protected, no matter where they may be. There are those who claim otherwise, but the fact is the truth. From the comfort of their homes to college and even in the streets They are all vulnerable to violence. Being in an environment where they can be attacked at any time at any time is extremely stressful for women. Let's consider the situation they face at work. Sexual harassment at work is a common thing in America.

Research has shown that the hospitality and food sector is the one with the highest number of these cases. It is followed by entertainment, retail and ten other legal fields. Another shocking research is the number of cases that are reported. This amounts to only 40% to 40% of total that occur. Many cases are reported, but many aren't. The root of the problem is due to the fact that women are not treated with respect and dignity. Women are exposed to snarky eyes, sexually explicit remarks, or even harassment sexually often at work location. There are a variety of strategies to address these situations. Women must first be aware of what constitutes sexual harassment and be aware of any incident that causes them to feel uncomfortable at workplace. Following that, they must know how to respond to the situation.

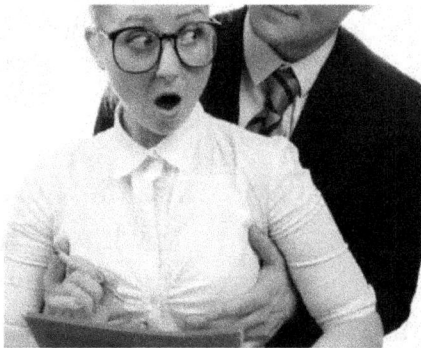

How do you define sexual harassment?

If a person working for you does not treat you with respect or sexually, in any way is a form of sexual harassment and is a crime. Making sexual remarks soliciting sexual favors, or touching you without your consent at any time is in violation of the law. It could involve anyone of any gender , and it is not restricted to males or women. It could be the perpetrator or victim. It doesn't matter who the harasser is, whether it's the employer, an employee, another employee or even a person who is not a associated with the business and is bound by the laws against harassment. If, at any time, an employee feels uncomfortable in her work environment because of her gender, and being subjected to physical or verbal harassing, she may bring a lawsuit against the harasser.

Things to consider when you aren't sure whether it's sexual harassment:

* Did the person's conduct made you feel uncomfortable? did you feel unwelcome?

* Did there occur any remarks that is sexual in any way?

* Did you notice any physical move that caused you to feel uncomfortable?

* Was it someone who holds a different position than you and threatened to interfere with your work?

Is the person's conduct negative to your performance and your mental well-being?

If the answer to all of these questions is yes, then it is time to raise it for sexual harassment.

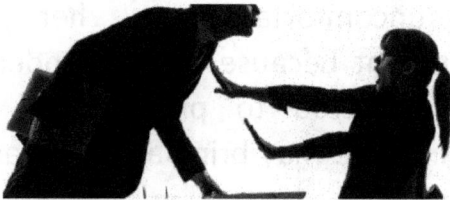

What can you do about it?

The first step is to stop these situations from ever happening at all. Employers must implement measures to make their workplaces a safe environment for everyone who works there. They must make it evident that everyone is at risk of being punished severely if incidents of harassment occur. If it happens then there must be an established procedure for how to handle it effectively.

Try to stay clear of engaging in a personal conversation or with anyone at work who make you uncomfortable or has an been branded as a misbehaving person.

First of all, women must be aware that they shouldn't be afraid to report the individual, regardless of what level of work he's at. Employers aren't legally permitted to punish those who file an allegation of sexual harassment. Therefore, every woman must know that they have the right to engage in a retaliatory action against these people at anytime.

Also, if the woman is uncomfortable with something even the smallest, she should express what they feel. Make sure that the person knows that their remarks or gestures aren't welcome. If the behavior is repeated or further taken you can ask someone who is trustworthy to look into it and file an official complaint. The first stage of the charge will be at the office or at a legal court.

Inform your employer and supervisor regarding the situation and file a formal complaint formal. Inform them about the incident and the actions you wish to take towards the individual who bullied you. Notifying them about it will help in court even if they fail to help out.

* Make it known and make sure that others are aware to ensure that the issue isn't buried or dismissed. Others employees may also assist to be witnesses or provide evidence later.

Speak to friends who are supportive and family members. Support groups can help you listen to those who have been through similar situations and how they faced the situation.

Make sure that the business investigates the incident thoroughly and take appropriate steps which are satisfactory to you. It is also important to ensure that the behavior does not repeated and you're not been subjected to the same harassment in the future. It could be that the person gets fired or sent to a different site. If the issue is not that severe it is best to have them properly disciplined and should not be required to further work with you.

* If the business is unable to take the necessary and appropriate action, start a legal case. The harassment is not just an unintentional touch or comment There are cases of rape, too. In these instances, take action and file the complaint immediately and notify the company , too. The prosecution of criminals will take place at an even higher stage.

How can we make work secure for women?

Every workplace or business should ensure that it is an appropriate place for women. There should be steps to stop any injury and also ways to take appropriate action against those who are in the wrong.

The process of educating people about what is acceptable and unacceptable can be the initial step. Everyone should be aware of exactly which behavior is appropriate and cannot be tolerated. The men should be aware that the company will take action strictly against any misdeed, while women are aware that they have the right to file a complaint when such incidents occur at any time.

A clear policy against sexual harassment is an absolute requirement at any workplace. It should be made available to all employees and strictly adhered to.

A committee is on hand to handle these complaints, investigate them and take appropriate step.

* The business can go above and beyond to help women learn the best way to protect themselves the case of any sexual assault, whether physical or verbal.

Chapter 6: How to Find The Evidence Of A Potential Crime

It is obvious that we cannot discern the thoughts of others. However, we can detect the body language and behaviour. What are the most obvious signs? A majority of criminals are guilty of something that is odd or suspect decisions before they commit the crime. Most of the time, this connects to the senses, as we discussed earlier. By gaining knowledge of these signals and recognizing them, we can increase our ability to spot any negative intents within us.

Rape: Rape isn't always an intentional act, and it is not always performed by strangers. It's not always easy to tell when compliments can quickly become your most terrifying nightmare. Do not fall completely under someone's attraction, particularly when you are attracted to them in a mutual way. Be aware of your safety to keep an eye on the situation and look for any strange behavior or indicators that indicate there could be another persona beneath the one that the person is portraying. In this instance you should trust your gut.

Stalk When you're in school you're likely to have the same schedule for the day. Be on the lookout for repeated "followers," someone who's always in the same place at all times. They could be following you, and is eager to learn your routine.

If you notice someone you suspect, stay away from them for a couple of days. If it persists more than that, you should change your route to see whether you can spot the same person. If you spot the person who is following you along the new route, consider this as a warning. Record the incident in your diary and notify the appropriate authorities right away. You might not want to cause a stir in the first place, but "it's safer to be safe rather than to be sorry" is a popular saying to a point.

Separate from Others: People with motivations to harm you tend to seek to separate you out of the crowd and separate yourself from your relatives and friends. They will always make up a variety of bizarre excuses or excuses to leave you isolated. Be cautious if you observe that this happens too often. If the person insists repeatedly to be alone with him an area, it could be considered to be a warning sign for danger.

Murder: In the case of domestic conflicts You should notify the police when somebody threatens to kill you during an argument. Other than domestic violence the majority of murders occur due to an armed attempted robbery. With regard to the earlier basic tips on avoiding going out at night, in dark areas and so on. It is best to be a victim of robbery attempts, if they occur. If you're confronted by a firearm and ordered to surrender money or valuables, such as purses, money and other items. It is recommended to hand over the item without reluctance in order to not risk your life.

Criminals tend to be scared when they are attacked they are frightened, and will often attack in response to opposition, and at this point the robbery can turn into murder.

Robberies: Robberies are more often being perpetrated by groups of people who work together. Be aware. For example, if you're leaving the supermarket and someone walks up to you in the parking lot and asks for directions, for a donation or a gift, etc. Be on guard no matter how innocent the person appears or how innocent the question. Criminals typically target the older or younger children to distract you as they take you by surprise from behind. A lot of carjackings happen in this manner.

The signs that precede assaults for the majority of crimes tend to be like. The perpetrator tries to take you off guard, frighten and then take over. Therefore, the most ideal situations are those where you're completely isolated and distracted. But that doesn't mean couples or friends out on their own aren't at risk of attack So everyone must be aware, even if you're not alone.

Violence: Be aware that you can learn a lot about the character of a person through their remarks as well as their suggestions, opinions, and reactions to a variety of circumstances. If you believe that a conversation is taking a negative direction, or that people participating in the conversation are becoming violent and aggressive, it should trigger an alarm.

There are some who purposely try to provoke other people, causing them to be a nuisance. This kind of person usually will try to convince you to start discussions about topics that you don't wish to talk about. They usually try to shame the other people around you or make mildly inappropriate remarks. In general, do your best to avoid those who are like this. People who are unhappy with their lives usually make it a point to cause problems in the lives of others. They will try to create misunderstandings--lies, misrepresentation of facts, influencing other people to become aggressive toward you and behave badly. Do not let this entice you into a rash reaction.

Remember, pick your battles. If you don't want someone to become violent with you, stay clear of being confrontational or engaging in confrontations verbally. To ensure your safety stay clear of these relationships in general.

Chapter 7: Warriors' Techniques, Mindset and Awareness

The most effective method of self-defense is to avoid. In order to be able to achieve this, you must improve and strengthen your awareness. Sure, it's good to beat an adversary in an open space, but know that in every fight you have a 50% chance of winning and losing could result in yourself killed. The best self-defense strategy is to be conscious of the surroundings around you and in a position to avoid the areas where conflicts are most likely to take place.

The Warrior's Tactic provides strategies to prepare your mind when you're out of your familiar zone. The mobsters will be there at the time you least expect them Therefore, your objective is to train the mind so that it is ready for any situation. The discipline and patience are the most crucial. Here are a few examples and strategies to completely avoid physical conflict:

While walking around the streets Make it a routine to keep an eye on the road once in a while. If you notice someone, look around to see what they wears or what he carries and also look at the form of his pockets and observe the form of his bulge. It is possible that he could be hiding something of weapon. It is not necessary to be looking at people in the eye. It is rude. It is only necessary to give him a only a brief glance or utilize an eye-to-eye.

If you spot the presence of a group of individuals a just a few feet away and they're walking to the exact opposite side to you, you should cross the street and stay clear of the crowd head-on. It is safer this approach, especially if they appear suspicious.

If you own a vehicle that is parked in a commercial zone be sure to check to see if anyone is in the car prior to entering. It will be a lot more difficult for a criminal to attack you when you are in your car, and you are unable to move around freely.

If you're driving and hit someone other person's vehicle (regardless the fault of who caused the cause) the first thing to do is ask whether the other driver is okay. This can help ease the tension of the incident and could even bring out an anger in the other driver.

If you're at an event and have to walk to the other area of the venue, you should not go through the middle or the center. You might see partygoers who are drunk and could get in troubles with them.

When you are sitting at the home of a family member make sure you sit in an armless chair. Place yourself on the opposite side of the couch so that you are able to get up faster in the event of having to. If you are sitting in the middle, and others are sitting on both your sides, it could be much more difficult stand up , particularly if you're in a self-defense situation.

There are syndicates that earn money by abducting people. They make use of a powder which, when inhaled can cause sleepiness and dizziness. In self-defense against anyone who is throwing powdered substances towards your face, you should keep your breath the longest time you can and get in the direction you are able from the area in which the powder was being thrown.

A typical human can keep his breath for twenty seconds, or even longer. So the possibility of escape shouldn't be an issue. Just do not let your assailant grab your hand. In the event that he is able to, take aim at the closest weak point on the bodies (refer the chapter on five) and then escape. In these situations it is not advised to grapple as you will have very little time to keep your breath. The best way to fight is with the longest weapon (whatever the limb is closest to your opponent) at the nearest important spot.

There are many methods to stay clear of a physical fight. However, there could be circumstances where you can't avoid fighting. In these situations it is imperative to be victorious because most street fights end once one is dead. Be aware, however, that your sole objective is to escape, and not end the life of. Doing self-defense too much and inflicting injury on the attacker could result in a backlash. He could bring allegations against you for injury. Even if you're defending yourself but the law will always prevail. If one hit is enough to let you go the law, do not take another step to follow it up with another.

A life-threatening situation is distinct from a normal self-defense scenario. In the event of a real danger to your life, then you're already able to employ lethal force that is capable of killing. One example is if three muggers in pursuit of you and are carrying weapons that are deadly, such as chains or knives. This gives you the right to defend yourself by using the most effective techniques. But, be prepared to prove before a judge the existence of a significant danger to your life and force you to kill or incapacitate the person who is attacking you.

The fear is present in all of us. Courage isn't simply the lack of fear. It is more about having complete control over your fear. You can utilize fear to your advantage however, it is important to note that this could result in your demise. If there's a danger to you, you'll be frightened. At times like this you go into the state of "fight or fight". If you decide to fight the fear of losing will transform to energy and make your strategies effective and your attacks harder. In contrast when you decide to fly your body may shake, and it will weaken. Make sure to work hard so that you can turn your fear into fighting force.

Chapter 8: Self-Defense Basics Strategies

These are self-defense techniques that anyone and everyone should be aware of. But, as a matter of precaution in case you skipped Chapters 1 or 2, you must go through them first. It is recommended to review some guidelines and rules prior to learning any strategies to defend yourself from an attacker. Basic principles like preventing an accident by being cognizant of what is happening around you and fighting as a final outcome should be among the first things to cross off your mind prior to thinking about engaging your opponent during a fight.

Do not punch your face. Make an eye Poke Instead.

Action films usually show heroes who punch the villain directly in the eye. It's cool and actually makes the hero appear like a powerful and unbeatable person. But this is only the case in films. In real life when you hit someone's face, you can expect your fists to cause injury quite a bit! It is possible to break your hand particularly if you've not been practicing.

Do you recall The Three Stooges? The old show which featured Curly, Larry, and Moe performing all kinds of slapstick and hilarious antics on the screen. One of their favorite jokes is an eye poke. Moe typically poking Larry or Curly in the eye and puts an end to their antics quickly. In reality the eye poke is an effective weapon for stopping an opponent than a direct punch on the face.

The newest fighter to win champion in the UFC's lightweight heavyweight division Jon "Bones" Jones is well-known for his fighting skills. In spite of his great fighting abilities however, there's one characteristic of his that has been accused of by majority of people who do not like him: he is known to poke at the eyes of his adversaries. A poke in the eye can deter even the most powerful person you've ever met.

However, if pokeing eyes doesn't appeal to you or you're worried that you'll miss your target, you can try scratching your eyes or hitting the eyes. You could even employ your knuckles for gouging the eyes of your adversaries. The most important thing is that you strike the eye multiple times. This is a very painful experience. It will cause your opponent to stop, take care of his eyes, shiver with pain or put his feet away and try to make his eyes to be clear. This will give you the time you need to get away.

Don't punch your face! Hit the nose using an open Palm

Another spot that's vulnerable on the human body is the nose. Also, kicking the face in hopes of hit the nose isn't always the most effective method of striking. If the attacker is directly in the front of you, and within arms's reach, an effective strike would be made using the palm's heel.

You must hit the nose with an upward straight motion with all your weight into the assault. If the person you are attacking is grasping you, take note that when you strike the nose, with all of your force, he'll release. It also gives the attacker another opportunity to strike. Repeat the strike when you can hit it as hard possible. If your attacker stumbles back or steps back to cover his nose, or squirms away in pain, then this is your chance to escape.

There are some who might be against this type of attack, saying that this attack is lethal. It is believed that one could kill someone using this type of strike because it could cause the bones to be pushed behind the nose upwards to the head. This is the same premise of the movie Con Air that starred Nicolas Cage. But, it's just an urban myth. The skull bones of skull so robust that they can't move regardless of the number of times that you strike the person in the face by striking him with your palm upwards.

Knife Hand Strike to target the neck

Another option that anyone could make is to strike the neck. Many people believe that you should strike at the throat of your attacker, however there's an even bigger target, which is the neck's side which is usually that is on the left side of your attacker (or the one that's within the striking distance of your right hand if standing directly in the front behind him). It's not a good idea to hit this side of the neck but you'll hit it, just like hitting an volley ball in the side by using your hand. This is referred to as the"knife hand strike. Keep your hands straight (not too straight, however) and ideally, tightly to each other. It is recommended to bend your thumb downwards to keep it from becoming overextended when you come in contact with the neck of your opponent.

The neck is where the jugular vein as well as the carotid vein are. If you strike it with enough force repeatedly, you could knock your attacker unconscious, albeit for a short time. But this gives you time to get away.

Knees, Kicks, Punches, as well as even slaps to the Groin

You've seen it a hundred times on television. Even the most powerful man on earth will collapse and cry in pain if they are hit by a the groin. If the attacker is male and is standing right in front of you , leaving the area unprotected, you can deliver an elbow towards the groin or just a quick kick towards the region of the groin.

When your adversary is trying to hold you back and you're within striking distance of the groin area, then hit this region (NOTE that the genitals are the most common area of attack since it's the one that is the most painful) or , if you are unable to hit him, just hit it as strong as you can, as often as you can.

Aims at the Knee

The knee is a major goal, and if you're aware of how to correctly execute a kick, it's another area to target. Later in this book , we'll discuss the correct way to deliver strikes, so we'll discuss the knee in the future. You can strike the knee from a variety of angles. If you hit your opponent's knees, he likely won't be able to catch your foot as it is too low. A knee injury can cause serious injury to your attacker, and may imprison him, offering you a better chance of escaping.

Everyday objects to use for self-defense

Even the things that you use on a daily basis can be used as weapons to protect yourself. This is especially useful when you're not in the same way as you were. In the event that you're in a parking spot and someone walks up to you, grab your car key and place it between your ring and middle finger as you create the shape of a fist. Naturally, the sharp end should stick out. This is the tool that you can use to scratch the eyes of your adversaries.

Even a magazine or newspaper could be used as a weapon that you can cut with. You can roll it tightly and fold the magazine into half. Punch on your foe with its folded side. The paper roll will be so heavy that it could fracture glass. A better option is an umbrella. If you don't want to strike your attacker in the face, attack your attacker in the arm with your umbrella (that is more efficient).

If you don't own mace, however you do have a bottle of hairspray, or perfume then spray it directly into the eyes of your attacker. If you're at the beach and being attacked, pick up the sand in a small amount and throw it on the attacker's face. Repeat the process repeatedly until some of the sand hits his mouth, eyes or the nose. The idea is to apply any object you can think of.

Chapter 9: What to Manage The Fear Factor

Imagine walking along streets in a risky zone at night, by yourself with a valuable watch and sneakers, a jacket, etc. You see an alleyway which is connected to the pavement. Are you crossing the street to stay clear of it? It is possible to walk faster to avoid any contact with the alleyway or anything else that might be on this corner. Or, simply stop. In this scenario, stopping and staying there is not the ideal choice. But, the idea of freezing might be appealing if you can hear some noises? Perhaps drunken yobs are coming toward you in the street. What do you do? What if they were the party-goers who came out after a night of fun?

The fear of the unknown can come up on us and make us think of the worst about the situation. It's because of an instinctual worry about what's next. The fear that we won't be able to handle this. I wasn't taught in this regard or taught how to behave or react in this scenario. The fear isn't of being out of control.

If you've never participated involved in physical confrontations, you're scared of the possibility of what could occur and how serious it could get. The thought of this is a thumping forefront of our minds. Then you sit in silence, which is precisely what the attacker is asking you to do.

To be clear, being hit is painful. The place you're hit will be based on the degree of intensity of the pain. The fact is that it's painful and unpleasant sensation. If you decide to not react then you're putting yourself at risk more than if you fight to defend yourself. The attacker isn't looking to be hit, and is likely to test your fear.

In such situations, it is essential to keep your head up. It sounds easy, but when you're afraid, it can be one of the most difficult things to accomplish. A steady breathing rate allows you to concentrate not on your fears but rather on the solution to conquer the fear. Being stifled by fear must provide you with the chance to figure out an escape route. In addition to finding an escape route you must break free from it. You can't be stifled by the dreadful scenarios you're facing.

Another way to combat anxiety is to begin moving. If you're stuck in fear, you're anticipating the inevitable negative. If you are able to keep moving, you're helping your body transfer your adrenaline from fear into action. It is basically preparing yourself up for whatever is thrown your way. It's like a fight workout. Everything that happens in the surrounding area, your sharp awareness of the surrounding and your well-balanced stance are prepared. That's not to suggest that you are able to defeat anyone who wants to cause harm to you in any way. However, this breathing and movement will assist you in getting over the fear of being in danger.

A lot of times, we feel anxious because we don't know how things will unfold. It is difficult to imagine any positive outcome from being confronted. Sometimes, this reasoning will ensure that we remain calm and safe from harm's way. When someone has determined that you're the one they want to target, slow down, bring your hands raised high with your neck and open palm. This is to protect yourself, while creating a barrier the front of you. The first step is to overcome the confidence you have in yourself. It is to manage anxiety. Continue to breathe. You're taking back control of your life instead of just waiting to see what happens. You are now prepared for the worst. You are thinking about backing down and trying to ease the situation, however, you are prepared to react.

Chapter 10: Traditional Martial Arts Techniques And Styles

After having gone over the basics, let's review some of the more classic fighting styles and techniques that have become popular across the world. Starting from Karate up to Krav Maga there is an unending array of styles and techniques to pick from. Each has its strengths and weaknesses. Here are a few of the most popular styles of traditional martial arts.

Krav Maga

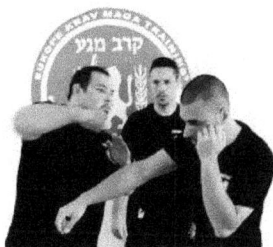

Krav Maga originates from Israel and has evolved into one of the most renowned martial arts. The Krav Maga fighting style is free of fancy gimmicks, and instead employs basic, yet effective techniques for full-body self-defense. The core of Krav

Maga is to protect yourself through any means needed.

Krav Maga adherents rain down punches at their opponents from close range to swiftly disable them. In this endeavor almost anything is allowed. That means that a punch to the shins, knees and even your crotch are all acceptable in this effective way of self-defense. The whole body becomes an effective weapon of force when you use Krav Maga, so don't be scared to utilize it!

Karate

The technique that is Karate has been practiced for a long time. It has only gained prominence in the West in the last 100 years or so, it has been refined over the course of countless generations. Karate is a method of fighting which employs jabs, slaps, chops and kicks. It's basically an all-in-one, non-armed way for self-defense.

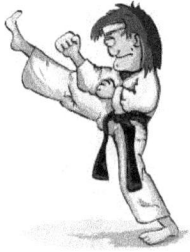

This is a perfect fit since Karate is actually one of the Japanese word, which literally means "empty hands". In the case of weapons, it is possible to be completely empty hands however it doesn't mean that you're invulnerable. Karate will teach you to make the most of the tools you have: your hands as well as your legs, arms and feet.

If you're shocked and unprepared by a crook on the street and you are not sure what to do, use your karate hand to put some common sense back at these criminals! It will definitely teach them the lesson of attacking others without prompting.

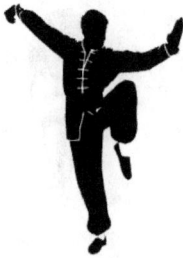

Kung Fu

The principal principle in Kung Fu is balance and form. Beyond just striking and kicks to an foe, Kung Fu specializes in fighting and controlling your adversaries. A skilled practitioner of Kung Fu is well versed with techniques such as flipping, throwing, and other ways of tackling an opponent.

In many ways , this makes it ideal for self-defense because a lot of the method in Kung Fu deals with mounting an attack. As anyone who is aspiring to become a Kung Fu Panda knows--this is an absolute recipe for success!

Muay Thai

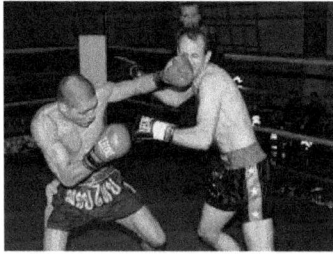

Muay Thai is mostly boxing, a type of sport that concentrates on specific upward strikes as in addition to stretching and tightening methods against the opponent. Muay Thai fighters aren't simply taught to strike with their hands but they're also permitted to utilize their knees, feet and shins in the most effective way and.

In Muay Thai you could hit someone on the head, then follow it up with an elbow on the face or leg to the stomach and then a quick kick towards the shins. It's the core of what gamers describe as an attack combination!

Simply, using your entire body to consistently pound an opponent, Muay Thai is certainly an element to be reckoned with. If you're looking for that additional security of learning a strong self-defense program, this type of martial art is an excellent place to begin your education.

Brazilian Jujitsu

Brazilian Jujitsu is yet another excellent form of martial arts that allows one to learn how to wrestle against an adversary. This method will teach those who learn it how to take control over a foe through using their own bodies weight to defeat them. If you are able to make use of the body weight of an opponent, you will be able to master the situation and make around in any direction, but remain loose.

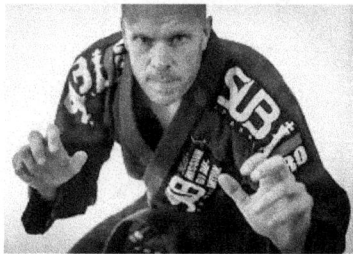

Through Brazilian Jujitsu, you'll learn to throw, flip, flip or otherwise nudge the aggressor until they are beaten to submission. If you are able to master this technique the more powerful they are, the harder they are - is definitely true. If you're in that situation, Brazilian Jujitsu just might be the right choice for you!

Chapter 11: Joint-Lock Self Defense

In the case of practicing self-defense, certain types naturally are more suited to the direct application when involved in an actual fight. In the case of joint-locks however, the way you training and actual experience are likely to diverge to a large extent. While you are practicing you and your partner, they will recognize that a joint-lock is approaching and be able to react accordingly this will not occur when you're fighting an adversary who is in the high of adrenaline, and always moving. Therefore, if you want to utilize a joint lock in a hand-to hand combat situation, you're likely to have to train and practice, then practise.

The most fundamental aspect of it is the Korean martial art of Hapkido where joint-locks play a key role in the practice, is about putting out the least amount of energy in every situation to effectively defend yourself throughout the time it requires. In other words, using joint locks as a means of defense, you should never take unnecessary effort trying to pull back from your adversary for the sake of locating an easier position to defend. This is due to the fact that moving away can be a type of aggressive behavior that can just result in more costs of energy, before all is over.

It is more efficient and , therefore, effective to protect yourself from the beginning by taking exact and precise actions. By doing this, you to to defend yourself quickly and gain an advantage that is unexpected while not letting the attacker know the strategy you have in mind to defend yourself.

Fundamentals of joint lock: To grasp the correct techniques for joint lock, you have to simply bend your fingers in the back of one hand. The pain this creates is amplified significantly by joint-lock methods. To comprehend how this could be effective in a battle scenario, imagine your opponent approaching you from behind and trying to strangle you. Instead of taking any other action, you simply take the attacker's hand with both your hands and then bend one finger back as much as you're able. Once you've got control of the finger of your attacker and you are able to determine any future actions or help them get on the ground by applying more pressure and directing their movements in the direction that you desire them to move in.

The main element that determines the efficacy of joint locks is moving the joint to the reverse to the direction it is intended to move. By manipulating the joint this manner, you take control of your opponent in a manner that is much more efficient than fighting against them directly in the majority of situations. Although it may not always be straightforward to initiate an effective joint-lock, the goal is to know what move will be most effective in the particular scenario, and then concentrate on striking an important weak point to get your adversary off guard enough to trigger the joint lock that you've selected.

The use of joint locks for targeting when deciding what kind of joint-lock will be most likely be the best-performing, the initial thing you'll be looking at is the kind of hold the attacker is currently able to exert over you. Nearly every joint of the human body is able to be secured and then controlled as it is the case that the appropriate circumstances are in place to allow it possible. So, when you are stuck by your attacker, the first thing you're likely to want to decide is the joints that are in easy reach and those that you can apply pressure to in the present situation.

Wrist joint lock The wrist is among of the joints that is easy to lock. To comprehend how this happens, the case, hold the wrist of your secondary dominant hand and push it back toward your forearm. This will result in a considerable amount of pressure and ultimately discomfort if you do not let go. Consider moving to the other direction, and move your wrist away from the arm and you'll feel another bout of discomfort. The numerous ways that the wrist is able to be adjusted makes it an ideal victim in many joint locking situations.

Mix strikes and joint-locks If someone grabs your shirt, the best method of controlling your situation is to hit them with the solar plexus. This will cause them to be stunned long enough to regain control of their hands. Simply by placing your thumb over upper part of their hand close to the middle and wrapping the remainder finger around your wrist, you've drastically changed the direction of the confrontation. You will then need to exert all of your force into turning the hand to the point that it's over the top, bent back toward the arm of the attacker while simultaneously bending it to one side.

With this joint lock it is not just ensuring that their grip on you is completely destroyed, but also induce them to be more cautious about their actions due to the discomfort they're in. You also make sure that there is nothing they are able to do as every single move they move will cause additional discomfort. When you're in this position, you are in all control over the attacker's movements. You could apply more pressure on the hold to bring them to knees or shift them in a different direction simply by pushing your wrist in the direction you want. You could even drop them to the floor by twisting your wrist more in any direction.

Neck joint-lock: If find yourself at the of a two-handed chokehold then the first thing that you will need to press down on your victim's groin, either using your hands or your feet, depending on which direction that you are facing. The next step is to grab their neck and pull your neck towards the left side with your hands that are dominant. bending upwards while using both hands. This will allow you to strength to turn your body away from the direction you are aiming for and then back toward the ground in an exercise that requires small upper body strength.

It is crucial to remember that making the effort to select the proper area to attack is crucial to this maneuver due to the manner in which you were attacked, the attacker's neck was left open. If the attacker is right in your direction, the neck is most likely to be a attack since it's hard to defend the neck and maintain an aggressive posture while at the same time. Therefore, you are able to quickly reach inside and hold the neck without the need to exert more energy in order to control it.

It is an attractive joint lock target as the musculature there isn't anything protecting it, therefore a single or double hand grab allows it to be pushed in the other direction easily. Once the neck is forced to move sideways, which is beyond its normal limitation, the spine is locked, and the attacker has no options other than what you would like to them to do. After that the manipulation and domination are a very simple and simple procedure.

Elbow joint-lock The elbow is yet another joint that is incredibly easily manipulated because, should your attacker grab you, there's bound to be a certain amount of distance between you and them. This distance is going to be bridged by arms, making the elbow a coveted and often vulnerable victim. It is possible to start by giving an upward chop to the elbow , which is often enough to release or break the hold completely.

In the next step, instead of pulling the hand back, you'll simply need to apply pressure to your elbow, while at the same time , bending the forearm against itself using the other hand. This will enable you to have instant control of the situation from either standing position or by causing your opponent to lower themselves through simply steering their bodies downwards.

If, however the attacker is grabbing you with only one hand, then you'll be able to raise your arm over the arm restraining you and place your arm below the joint of your elbow. The attacker will have two options, either release their grip on you, or keep the grip, and lock not just the elbow, but their entire hand and arm completely secured. After the lock is completed, the attacker has no decision to make and you will be able applying pressure in order to raise them up while they attempt to lessen the pain. This leaves the attacker open to a quick kick to the legs that could result in them falling to the ground swiftly.

Chapter 12: What to Do and Do Not!

Remember that crime is possible because it is possible that it could occur to anyone, anyplace and at any time! So , be aware! Beware!

The different in the cultural practices of a country could be the different ways of life of people. What is their relationship and dress? This turned into one of the most important elements along with the crime of rape, as there's the possibility of.

The most recent case study has found that 73 % of rape crimes are that are committed by those you know as acquaintances, new friends or neighbors, and even family members so being aware of your environments is imperative.

You must now learn to be alert to your surrounding environment. You must be taught to guard yourself against other people. Learn your child at an early age about how to defend themselves when they are people who are causing trouble them. Remember! Children are also at risk of sexual assault, not just girls, but also boys. They are so cruel! Do not allow them to be a part of your family.

DO!

1. Make sure you lock your door while you sleep.

In the night, we wouldn't know what was happening Many murders, robberies and even murders occurred while the victim was asleep. To guard yourself from happenings that you do not want to be around, we must lock the bedroom door before going to bed. The bedroom is a private space therefore you must not let anyone in without permission. establish a routine.

2. Lock your door.

Sometimes , when we're exhausted we forget to secure the doors. ensure that you secure the door you're sleeping or even during the day when you're on your own. Since rape doesn't just occur at night, but it can happen even during the day.

3. Secure your home with alarm as well as Closed Circuit Television (CCTV)

If you reside in a city that is crowded the alarm system and CCTV are an absolute requirement. You can regulate the environment outside your home with CCTV and alarms to provide warning should someone attempt to gain access without your authorization.

4. Set the tools of self defense in strategic locations.

This is a way to safeguard yourself in the home. Set the items that you can defend yourself in strategic areas like bedrooms, living rooms and the kitchen, family room, or even near doors or windows as the moment you press, it will be simple to use these tools. The tools you could employ include a stun tool insect spray, blow-rounders the pepper spray and so on.

5. Have a weapon of self defense whenever you leave your home

Make sure to have a self-defense tool with you whenever you leave the home, it's a small tool that you can put into a pocket or bag and has many advantages. Tools you can utilize to protect yourself from criminals includes scissors and bullpen, a miniature stun tool, and perfume with a form similar to the bullpen is also useful and is available for selling at the stores and you can also carry a pepper bottle that you make using pepper powder and water. Once you have it in the bottle. It is small enough that spraying it in the eyes of the criminals to make him lose his focus and you'll protect your self.

According to the most recent statistics of rape crime, it occurred between 06:00 and 18:00, at a rate of 33 percent. This is in contrast to the fact that they happens at night just 24 percent, so be cautious during daylight.

10 rapes take place in the home of the victim, however only 2 of 10 instances of rape happened at the residence of relatives, friends, or acquaintances of victims . one of 12 instances of rape was in a parking lot. In certain countries, rapes is also a common occurrence in public transport like in India when rape was committed in public transport. The victim was killed and the body was thrown onto the road. In Indonesia there have been rapes on public transportation, and in taxis. with robbery.

It is possible to avoid this from happening by not using public transportation in case the car is the quiet, or there are just a few males without female passengers, as they may be part of a be a rapist group. Don't also take public transportation with black glass so that passengers who are not inside the vehicle can't observe the condition that you are in inside the vehicle. If you are taking a taxi, check that the taxicab the registered name isn't an illegal, and make sure you have you have the driver's ID card and, if needed it is necessary, examine the trunk of the car and make note of any vehicle that you are in and then give it to your family or friends who believe that should something happen to you, could be easily tracked by family members or your family.

It is not advisable to travel on public transport alone. You was immediately disapproved of by the driver when he said that the road was not running like normal to reduce traffic congestion or to speed up the travel time. When you realise that you're traveling on several roads, you are soon called for help via your mobile phone to the police or a trusted friend. There are other rules to follow. Do not rest while on public transportation , and be alert!

DON'T!

1. Don't wear too tight and sexy clothes

People dress to be shorter and wide-legged is regular or normal, but to dress for short-skirted attire, such as going to school or to the supermarket. Do not wear too short, which is the reason for this is because it may cause immorality or even sexual rape. God designed the female body in all its splendor and beauty, so how can you not preserve the beauty of your well-being of the body and are devoted to your husband, who you have all of your body.

2. Do not update your status of your social media accounts while you're in a private space

One tool for sharing quick information is social media like facebook, twitter and many more. You can connect with other people around the world , and you can also transmit any information. However, sometimes we forget that there are certain information can be shared with others and it is no reason to share it. One example is to tell anyone else that you are at home by yourself and you are using social media, as you don't know the identity of the people who are followers or friends on your social networks. until now, the murder and rape also took place on social media.

3. Don't use excessive jewelry.

Avoid wearing jewelry that is too large while outside of the home, for example, when you attend an event. Many instances were triggered by robbing, attackers who staged the next crime, namely rape. Avoid making use of mobile phones when in public places.

4. Don't wear high-heeled shoes.

If you leave the house , you can only wear heels, especially for professional women who require stylish attire with high heels. However, you shouldn't wear high heels when coming home from work in the evening You can wear flat shoes after you return home. It is helpful in the event of situations that require you to be running at the speed of light.

5. Don't exaggerate.

Be aware of your body language and stay clear of excessive behavior when speaking to strangers because body language may be inviting them to do something to you. Be sensible, don't be appear arrogant or confident and avoid getting in too much contact with strangers. There are many other things that shouldn't be done and ought to be taken care of to stay clear of sexual exploitation and other immoral actions. It is essential to increase your awareness and emotions is to also apply your reasoning, as women generally have strong opinions about what's about to occur.

Chapter 13: The Weaknesses Of Human Anatomy

Understanding the weak spots in your body are is crucial for a successful attack as well as an escape. The objective is to eliminate the attacker , and knowing where his weak spots are is only helping you more. If you find yourself in a battle it's useless to continue to pound your opponent, or launching in a blind way with punches and kicks. You'll only waste your energy and time and will make you tired more quickly.

Use your opponent's weakest places to gain

A hook that is inserted into the jaw- A quick and strong blow to the front of the jaw can be quite surprising to snap a person's neck! This useful move could result in death instantly.

Inflicting damage to the Adam's Apple- one quick and abrasive hit at the Adam's Apple region can result in the crushing of the windpipeand blowing out the entire wind of the attacker, and making it extremely difficult for him to breathe.

Afflicting a rage on the Templesand threatening temples on your forehead , on either side, could be fatal to someone in a matter of minutes. It's a tiny bundle of nerves and massive blood vessels, all tied inside the temple.

Stamping the small of the BackA solid punch, stamp or elbow strike on this region can cause spine injuries that are both severe and minor based on the severity of the strike. Most often, this causes immediate death.

Do not nick the Nasion. Simply hitting the nasion with your finger or hammering it over time will heal. If you truly want to take down your attacker and force him to pay for all the crimes he committed make sure you put your bat in the nasion, the most well-known cartilage region in the brain. In this way, he'd certainly have compensated for his crime!

Cerebellum's Base- an intense and swift strike to the beginning of the spine, which is the area beneath the skull may result in immediate injury or even death.

Doing a smack on the testicles. A extremely powerful blow to the testicles can be extremely painful which can trigger. If it isn't causing death, it is likely to reduce your adversary to his knees.

Take the time to feel the philtrum. Grab one of your fingers and put it the middle of your nose, and lip. The fragility of this is one of our body's weaknesses. Since it's full of nerve endings, it's an extremely easily targeted to attack.

Kick the CoccyxThe tailbone is a bony structure that if you kick it in the middle and then in an upward direction is enough to fracture it. The forceful shock to the spine itself can be fatal.

Hit the Heart- A forceful punch at the heart in one quick motion could crush your heart! You'll need to be robust to be able to deliver an effective punch.

Punches to the underdog - this type of punch can cause necks to snap upwards direction. A single blow coming at you from below can be sufficient to be fatal.

The Full and Half NelsonAttack the attacker from behind, and then wrap your arms around them as if you were taking them in a hug. While doing this you should push your arm upwards , while moving your hands toward to the peak of your heads. This will allow you to move your head forward, and break their neck in the entire process. When you are in the half-nelson your only arm can be used to stop the attacker's hand from performing another attack.

Stomach Stomach PainA punch that is landed in the pit of your stomach and the gut could result in damage to important organs in the body. Sometimes, the impact could be powerful enough to cause the state of organ dysfunction.

Straight into the Rib Cage - attacking the rib cage may cause pain that is severe but also damage lungs or other organs which can lead to deathly organ and body complications.

The brain is busted. This is a powerful technique that is a good option if are caught in the middle of a battle with the concrete. Gran onto the belt or loop of jeans of the opponent and lift him up and then fall backwards on your back. This could result in them smashing into the concrete, and then hitting their head against the concrete along the sides which causes a slamming of the neck, and other serious issues.

Wall punch: backing your opponent against the wall, and launching a punch at him could break and smash his windpipe , and even slash their neck.

Head yank: If you hit the head of the attacker first to the side, the remainder of the body is immediately weak and slack. The best method for doing this is to press against the chin, and then make an jerky movement. If this isn't holding him in place for long enough, smack your eyes, or poke at the soft flesh inside the nose, too.

Head concussion- one strong strike to the head of your adversary that is placed against a wall could cause a severe head injury or, in the case of a strong punch, the punch could result in the breaking of the skull!

Choke Slam - not like the well-known WWF move, you simply wrap your arm tightly around the throat of the attacker. When you exert enough pressure, you will be able to smash their windpipe and break their neck.

Eyes are an easy target that can cause hurt if they are swung by fingers. If you're being held or groped, simply reach your hands at the attacker's face using your fingers or an pointed object and strike the attacker in the eye. A punch that is sufficiently hard will cause enough pain , and your eyes begin to swell and cause pain, not letting the attacker to watch you flee. Just bringing your hands closer to his eyes can cause him close them by reflex and give you the time to hit the attacker or kick him.

Do the tooth if you're being pushed down and you have your hand restrained, your teeth could save you. Simply bite his ear, which can be the most painful thing, or whatever else that falls within your reach. Make sure you bite hard enough that it is bleeding and causes your attacker sufficient pain that they temporarily let go of you.

The head or throat with a weapon that is hard could cause pain, causing injuries and death for the victim. If the assault is a life or death scenario, a counter-attack like this is generally not needed. If you're confident that you are able to stun the attacker or make him blind for a time and then escape or escape, then you should go for this option.

The groin area in the torso area is one of the areas that are most vulnerable for both genders. A knee strike or punch that is just powerful enough could cause serious injury. If you're thrown to the ground and are able to touch the attacker's stomach by punching, take a shot at it.

Twisting the wristThe wrist is an easily accessible area that can be injured. If you're carrying an racquet or stick as well as a club ensure that you hit it with a sharp force on your wrist, the upper part of your forearm or even the side of your waist. All of these are likely to make the attacker weak and will permit you to escape.

Hands that are a bit painful- Hands are among the first items attackers grasp. The fingers of an attacker as well as the fingers on the opposite side may be bent reverse direction or stretched wide enough in order to cause severe pain, and even disrupting grip. If you're not extremely skilled do not try any hand lock because it could be detrimental in the event that you fail to make an effective attempt.

The feet contain sensitive points that can be tapped to deter your attacker. If you're stiletto-wearing, then you could go into his feet and cause him to suffer severe discomfort.

Chapter 14: Martial Arts And Self Defense

Which martial art is the best to use for Self Defense?

A number of frequently asked questions about self-defense is what martial art is the most effective to defend oneself. It is a big subject that is going on. In reality If you ask many martial arts masters across the world today , each of them will be arguing on the particular style they have learned.

If you're talking to someone who is a mixed martial artist, they will be arguing for the art have been mastered by him. It appears as if every master is advocating their own style. Mixed Martial Arts (MMA) attempts to solve this issue by contrasting different forms of art against each other. This is a worthy endeavor that ultimately led to the evolution of styles that's what that we are witnessing now.

Combat art practitioners are referred to by various styles, examples of which include mixed martial artists free style fighter and so on. But, despite the intermixing of these martial arts, it is not enough to solve the basic question of what martial art is most effective for street defense or for real-life defense.

MMA is now an activity that is governed by rules and equipment that safeguards both the fighters and their equipment. It is the same when trying to match an art of fighting against another form of combat in a casual encounter. There are rules that regulate the contest. These rules are designed to ensure that the sparring sessions are fair. These rules also offer an extra layer of security for the combatants as well as for.

That's the biggest drawback of the entire process. It is because when you are in the real world of self-defense, there aren't any rules. If a man (or many males in many instances) is threatening to confront you, they will not comply with any laws. There will not be a judge to end the fight if one of the participants falls to the ground and is left helpless.

Therefore, it's almost impossible to decide which one is the most effective one there. Every combat art has its own strengths (that's certainly the case) and all also has weaknesses and weaknesses (that's certain too). There are specific aspects of every fighting art, which are applicable to street combat.

Since not all techniques can be utilized by an ordinary civilian, the best option is to study the ones that work in the street and employ the techniques that anyone could do. There may not be the time or energy to become a self-defense weapon, but you could spend the time to master specific techniques that will assist you in stopping any attacker who might try to attack you. You don't need to be a black belt through two to four martial art forms (that could take years!) But you can study specific techniques you can employ to protect yourself.

Self-Defense vs. Martial Arts vs. Sports Fighting

This section will shock you to the core. When UFC was still a young sport and the Ultimate Fighting Championship was still in its early stages (UFC 1 through UFC 5), the people in general only knew about the stand-up fights that were popular as well as striking art. That's thanks to marketing initiatives of the mass media.

They didn't know about Brazilian Jiu Jitsu (BJJ) the art of grappling that concentrates on combat with the feet. This is the reason Royce Gracie won 3 Ultimate Fighting Championship tournaments (UFC 1, UFC 2, and UFC 4). Some have described him as an "human anaconda. When he grabs grip on you, you're gone.

BJJ and the other mixed martial arts community is constantly evolving, always evolving, and always growing. But, it doesn't alter the fact that it's still an activity. Even if you are involved in fighting sports, that does not mean that you are

106

proficient in self-defense. Keep in mind that self-defense and martial art aren't the same thing. It is possible to be 6-degree BJJ black belt, just like Royce Gracie but it is not a guarantee that can protect yourself from a emergency situation in which the life of you (or your life and that of other people) is at stake.

Combat sports and martial arts will provide you with a decent workout and keep you in good shape. This is a crucial aspect of life, and is a great asset when you need to defend yourself against the threat of an attacker. But the combat sports and martial arts are designed for young and physically fit individuals (i.e. those who are athletic). They are based on rules, that means you're drilled and taught to play by the rules while your adversary does not have any rules, he'll attack and hack whatever way he wants.

Self-defense strategies are able to be learned and applied efficiently even by elderly, weak and frail. It is possible to be in poor fitness or older but you still have the ability to be a master of self-defense. As we mentioned earlier, it can take years to master martial art. Self-defense abilities however, can be learned much quicker, sometimes within a matter of weeks or even months.

Self-defense that is street style also has no limits. There aren't any restrictions, and you'll learn to defend in ways not permitted in combat sports. Self-defense will put your mentality at the same level as the attackers, however your goals will differ. Your attacker may be motivated by intention while you, on the other hand, are fighting in order to get out of the way and remain secure. It's kinda altruistic, however, it's also true.

The similarities between Martial Arts and Self-Defense

But both self-defense and martial art share a few things in the same. These similarities prompted some forms of martial arts to transform into real self-defense art. These similarities are primarily related to the practical application of combat arts in real-world situations.

Self-defense and martial arts techniques can help you become familiar with your physical capabilities and limitations. They will train you in specific skills that can assist you in protecting yourself from physical assaults. They will show you how to be conscious of the surroundings, and how to prevent any form of assault, abuse and even attacks from happening at all. They will also help increase your self-confidence. Both of them will strengthen the connection between your body as well as your mind.

Chapter 15: Learn Spiritual Cleansing

Synopsis

Conducting a cleansing for the spirit of someone else is a difficult job to accomplish. It takes more focus and it is necessary to plan all the necessary preparations prior to when you begin the process. Spiritual cleansing isn't intended to replace any form of medication or treatments. However it is an effective tool that you can utilize to maintain both your physical and spiritual well-being. It will be possible to attain this if you regularly use it. All you have to do is gather all the ingredients you need, search for an area where you will be able to do this effectively and be ready to bring clarity and health to the life of someone else.

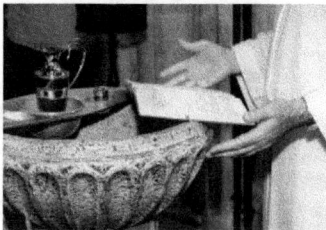

Steps to Cleansing

Here are the steps you must follow to achieve a positive spiritual cleansing effect:

1. No matter what location you decide to work in for the task, be sure that you've got it ready prior to when someone with when you arrive. Clean the area and free of impurities by cleaning and dusting. Make a sage stick into a smoke and, when it's lit blow it out and let the calming smoke mix with the air moving through the corners of the room. Smoke can assist in identifying the places in the room where positive vibrations are present.

2. Consider and take the time to cleanse your aura and then align your chakras prior to beginning the process of cleansing your spiritual energy. Relax on a seat and put your eyes shut while you concentrate on the positive energy you feel. This is vital because you need to remain positive during the process.

3. Make sure your friend is prepared to go through the spiritual cleansing. Place him/her on a mat. Ask them to shut their eyes. Breathe slowly in order to help them relax and be focused for an entire cleansing. Make sure that the person is at ease and comfortable. After that, instruct the person to pay focus on the breathing throughout this spiritual purification. Keep your mouth shut and refrain from talking while you are doing the cleansing.

4. Cleanse, then gently fluff your aura around the individual using your hands. Keep both your hands of the left and right hand at 6 inches from the body of the person and focus on the energy that the person has. Beginning at the head, move your hands in the air until they reach his feet to draw out the negative energy. You can do this by making gripping movements with your hands. It is not necessary to contact your body so you can get rid of the negative energy. The next step to do is request your friend to lay down and after which you repeat the same action again.

Then, you can fluff your aura by using both sides of their body using broad movements across the whole body, without touching them.

5. Cleanse the negative energy from the body of the individual beginning with the head all the way to the feet. Make sure to eliminate the negative energy completely. Try to feel the aura of the individual, then wipe the person's aura using your hands beginning at the front and moving all the way to the back of the body. This will assist the body get rid of the negative energy that persists after the cleansing exercises that you have done.

6. Find the hot and cold areas of the body. Focus on the warmth of all areas of their body. Start with the head and continue until you get to the feet. If there are any body parts that are hot, try to radiate coolness and healing using your hands, pointing at the body. Then, begin to transfer of energy. Begin by shaking hands in order to remove the negative energy on

the hands. Once you have done this, your process is done.

Chapter 16: Home Invasion (Break-In)

The violation of immunity to residence[12] refers to the fact that an individual visits a person's home or any of its buildings (garden garage, garden, etc.) without consent or is unable to exit after having been admitted with consent in accordance with the Penal Code of Turkey.

In the first place, it is important to know that "you are not required to open the door for anyone who calls!" Unless you have set up an appointment or an earlier phone call or you're expecting someone to visit, anyone who knocks on your door is not a stranger. When you do decide to knock on the door, it is important to perform a situational evaluation according to "awareness" which is an essential thing to be aware of always. First, look via the eye. If you notice an unknown person and you have to open the door for a reason, exchange the items using the safety latch or the chain that is attached to the door. If you have to open the door a bit more then please shut the door when you go back to your home, bring cash, or other items. Bring the change , then reopen the door.

What to do in the event of a home invasion or break into are covered within the chapter "SKILLS and PLANS".

IN SUMMARY: Awareness:

Do not let anyone get in your personal space.

Make sure you are managing contacts that are not yours.

Always do an assessment of threats.

Be more cautious if are in transitional areas

Be prepared for dogs[13or any other animal attack. Focus on running away and hiding instead of fighting them.

ATTITUDE AND A MANNER

Our manner of conduct and attitude, i.e. behaviour patterns to defend ourselves and ourselves at the beginning of our journey to self-defense are important following an awareness phase. The steps to be taken in an argument over traffic rights of way or line-jumping, or parking space disputes are different from those used for pickingpocketing, robbery or abuse.

Ability to communicate and calm

If you recognize the possibility from an assault, this is a sign that the threat or attack has already occurred or already been able to enter into your private space. As an example, suppose that the situation is an argument over parking spot or a position in a line. The best course of action is to not escalate the conflict regardless of whether you're correct, and to get control of your self-esteem and keep it from driving you into a rage. These are essential "Abilities to calm". Do not get involved in "Ego battles" with criminals with guns[1414]. The majority of fights revolve around an individual's ego[15[15,16]. Don't try to keep pace on the Joneses. This is not only about your words, but also your body language. Control your ego[16]. Avoid infuriating others with your words, gestures or imitations. In particular, refrain from touching in any manner! Don't start any fight with an arm-wielding or knife-wielding robber , or any other pedestrian in the traffic.

Even if you're right and strong There is no definitive winner in a fight or dispute. Speak up and say "I'm sorry, I'm sorry and you're right when the fact" before any serious or tragic outcomes occur. If you're confronting an uninformed or ignorant person. You must plan to end the discussion in the most efficient and fastest manner in a short time. This is known as "Verbal skills" also known as "Verbal Judo" that is a separate science. It is a science that is essential not just to protect yourself but in every aspect of your life, including business wedding, school, and marriage.

A loss in judo verbally escalates into a physical loss[17The physical loss can be a result[17. One must be aware of an attack in the verbal exchange and avoid striking with a sudden force. People who are smart, however are usually in a disadvantage because of their defensive posture because the person who is attacking decides when the attack will occur. We only know the signs of attack, and then attempt to escape or avoid. This case is explained in section "Pre-Attack Indicators/Pre-Attack Cues". Maintaining your defensive posture is defined in section "MARGIN as well as DISTANCE".

Participatory Verbal Judo

We must choose to adopt actions and attitudes that work equally physically and mentally as our bodyguards and protectors and also contribute to that in terms in terms of our body language, at whatever point of verbal Judo. Also calm and soothing posture is required like putting your hand(s) up in the air with palms open, declaring "Okay, easy...I don't wish to do any harm or cause harm to you." ..." This form of body language is described in the section on Defensive Fences/Defensive.

Participatory verbal judo can be used when you abide by the attack and are able to plan the chance to counterattack and also bears the traces of your reluctance or adjustment to the attacker. Verbal judo break the ice by saying things like "okay but not hurt me, I are able to take my entire cash". Be aware and constantly try to use your brains to take advantage of the opportunity to counterattack. escape or come up with an idea.

"Keeping calm and cool[18Staying calm and cool[18" when it comes to physical or verbal fights is the primary and difficult part of protecting ourselves and our loved ones from any threat. It is essential to learn to avoid engaging in fights and to develop a sound strategy during a fight, or to recover the losses incurred after an attack is essential. These subjects will be further discussed in the following parts of the text.

Pre-Attack Indicators/Pre-Attack Cues

If verbal judo gets more aggressive and fights escalate, pay attention to your "Signs that indicate a Fight." You must be particularly attentive to his eyes because the eyes are the windows to the soul. Also, you should watch his hands - they are the windows to intentionsand head/shoulder movements to identify whether an attacker is looking for an opportunity to strike above or in front of him. "Pre-Attack Indicators "pre-attack indicators[19]"need to be carefully read. Never ignore pre-attack cues. The attacker's attempts to keep his hands from your view or drop his gaze to the floor (getting ready to punch) are considered an indication of a possible punch that could be thrown on your face or a knife that will be stabbed through your body. The waist, hands and eyes are all pre-attack indicators. Be aware of your shoulders to determine the movement of hands.

Underestimation

If you meet someone, regardless of his gender, age, or physical condition beware of his physical or mental condition! Don't fall into"the "normalcy prejudice." No matter how weak an attacker appears to be, it's quite likely that you will be stabbed or have your face exposed to chemical agents by an uninvited person at an unpredictably moment. The fear of being in danger can weaken the actions, behaviors, and attitude that are needed to guard against this type of danger. Never underestimate a potential tragedy!

Deathly Force Encounters at the Speed of Light

Let's say that there's an immediate attempt to harm property or lives or it's an instance of violence. In the event that the attacker directs a punch at us, we would be unable to think of how massive "the speed at which deadly forces encounters[20[20,21]". In the normal flow of daily life, someone could unleash a punch from an outburst of anger. A knife could be stabbed quickly and abruptly...A quick hit upon a painful area on your body could be enough to kill you and leave you in a state of unconsciousness like a hidden knife that was pulled out in a flash could cause your death after a few tens of a succession of slashes.

Even if you own a firearm and the attacker is carrying knives (assuming you are sure that your gun isn't aimed at the attacker, but is in the concealed holster) the attacker will likely beat the gun (your firearm) by using the knife. This is an interesting , but scientifically proven fact that is referred to in"the "Tueller Principle". It's an interesting reality that the knife has the upper hand over against a firearm. A person who is armed with a knife may reach a distance of 21 feet (6,4 meters) and then stick his weapon in front of the police are able to shoot at the targets. It can be done within 1.5 minutes. Even if the person who is threatening to attack you has been shot by the gun, a knife could be already wounded into the police. Police usually perform a formal training session on rapid draw, aiming and shooting as well as exercises to draw away and place the objects (such as tables, boxes and boxes.) between the attacker and him, creating barriers.

Bystander Effect/People Around

Be aware that you're all alone at the time of attack. There won't be anyone nearby to defend you, and others around are likely to be largely bystanders who might be astonished or be afraid to speak up or think "who really cares, let them at it" and then walk away (this approach is correct in certain ways. This is further explained under the section "To Step In to Step In" or Not to Step in"). If you're on your own with the attacker, all you hold is your mindset and spiritual skills and tools for defense, as well as your wisdom and strategy.

The Bystander Effect is broken

Let's say you're being targeted. You are feeling like you're unable to deal with the situation on your own capabilities. The situation gets more difficult however, no one is bothered or just watch the situation go by. What do you do? Here's the solution Break the effect of bystanders[2222. That is, contact someone for help , but what is the reason and what?

There are two motives one of which is easy to figure out. Since you're in trouble and it's becoming worse and the clock is ticking. You must contact witnesses and collaborate with them in order to save yourself or other victims. The third argument is that in the event that it is possible to manage to survive or overcome the attacker and injure anyone else by using the techniques described under the heading "SKILLS and PLANS" You will have to prove your case by bringing witnesses to your side and recording cameras there for you to comply with legal guidelines and laws. [23]

How can we contact bystanders to assistance? The answer can be found in the section titled "Distractions". But, remember that even if help is offered but it is not immediate! The worst thing is that it won't arrive. Be mindful of Allah and keep in mind to pray.

Chapter 17: Training

The second thing we must consider is how to prepare for real attacks. In the present, we live be living in a world full of quick solutions for every problem. The truth is, there isn't anything as an instant fix.

The notion that everything happens in a flash is not the case. In fact, the way that people live their lives does not reflect reality. Constantly eating, without considering the expense of having to pay for their purchases.

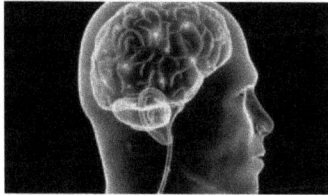

We must first develop a habit. This means paying close attention to the things we are learning. Training carefully! Martial Arts are after all "body mental and spiritual."

For many people in our day and age, it's all about the body!

The average person is thought to have 70k+ thoughts every day. It is a problem that the majority of these thoughts are negative! Is there any surprise that there are many problems? The subconscious mind will be convinced of everything you say. It is especially true of those things we say through our imagination.

There's a saying that says seeing is believing However, there is plenty of evidence that believes are seeing! Below, I have linked an article about how effective this technique could be!

So , what are you doing during your martial arts education? It's time to return to the basics! Make sure you turn off any distracting devices. Music is an amazing thing, but it requires an uncluttered mind to be able to train! It is common to listen to music in dojos to help promote the training. It's fine for training that is aerobic however, not for self defense! You need to be able to concentrate and be able to visualize what's taking place!

Let's take a look at possible steps to achieve this during training, and backed with visualisation.

Traditions play a crucial part in this training, however today we are often not interested in the things that have been proved to be effective!

Kata training is vital! It allows you to develop balance, movement and coordination. Additionally, it gives you the chance to observe self-defense applications by using your imagination! It's not real however it doesn't need to be. It is a great way to help teach the response to certain movements and transform fine motor skills useful! Kata can teach a variety of things however, only to those who is also willing!

* Self Defense techniques. They are also great for long since they're executed with focus and focus!

Doing the same thing over and over is not going to be effective. Like in Kata! Kata! The actions must be mastered before the speed needs to increase until move becomes more like real-life speed. It is recommended that when the levels rise that "talk" be integrated into the lessons! It can be a problem for concentration in an Dojo but special arrangements are made to allow this! I've even taught students who are in darkness and do not know who is fighting! Do your best to make self-defense training easy and efficient! Yes multiple techniques is possible and must be utilized! Keep it simple! Complex

Techniques can be enjoyable however, the realities of life often don't go according to the way we think they should. The mind has to be trained to react to the events that occur, and not just following a pattern.

Play around! Take on different distances, with different punches , and various attacks. At the top level, have the student be able to respond to what's happening, not what or she anticipates to occur! When the mind is completely engaged , the results will be evident.

If this is coupled with visualization , even when outside of the Dojo the magic starts to take place!

Here, I'm going to mention that this kind of training that is intense can be very frustrating and requires require some time! Thus, visualization as well as strong support and encouragement from your instructor is essential! It is normal to be frustrated, but not letting it go will cause failure and weaken your work from Chapter 1.

The Experience is changing

When you are done with the course, you must deal with the mistakes you have made. The best thing you can do is to laugh about them and have fun doing it. But, the best way to rectify the above is to take at least 10 minutes replaying the experience, but changing your reactions into picture flawless responses! The more you practice this, the better you'll do during physical training!

Personal example: When I started my training in 1984, I realized that I was somewhat scared of breaking wood in preparation for an exam for belts. At the beginning, I watched my first grade as higher belts tried and frequently failed to make these breaks. I didn't want to become someone who made it high and fell! Therefore I began to envision going through all the breaks that took me from Green Belt through Black Belt in perfect form! I could imagine hearing my instructor tell me how to proceed, as well as I could hear the applause when I successfully performed the procedures. What did I do? I was in the same place for 10 years without missing any break! including aerial kicks and bricks.

Visualization is a great tool!

The Habit of Creation

Here's a challenge to you! You need 21 days in order to alter an attitude, or break an old habit. It requires 21 days in order to develop an entirely new habit! Try this method in 21 days! Absolutely no Negative thoughts, or complaining!

If something happens to you, take a moment to stop it and eliminate it from your life! Accept the situation and then rectify the behaviour with positive action! Within the next 21 days that your life will be better! It's really that easy!

Establishing good habits is crucial to be successful in any endeavor! People want a well-organized, disciplined lifestyle with enough chaos to make it enjoyable. To be successful in self-defense, you must take time each day to practice contemplation as well as exercise! However, I'm hearing the excuses right now. "I do not have the enough time." What this really means is that you don't want to! However, don't worry! The fact is that the 16 hours the average person stays in a state of alertness is mostly unproductive.

In most offices, where employees are working for eight hours daily, only 2 hours is productive! What is the amount of time you spend, and I'm talking about social media platforms like Facebook?

I had a student that trained in a frenzied manner for five years in order to achieve the rank of first Dan Black Belt. After achieving this goal, I started to notice missed class and explanations of poor attendance. In reality, is that "failure" method of my unconscious mind started to take over, and eventually TV was more important than the training! All it came down to bad thought!

If you don't perform the job, who else will? If you're not trained to safeguard your life, do you think that the police will show up and help you?

Chapter 18: Before The Fight

Intuition

In the previous chapters , we examined the preparations for diverse kinds of dangers and threats. The focus of this chapter is on events that lead up to the confrontation.

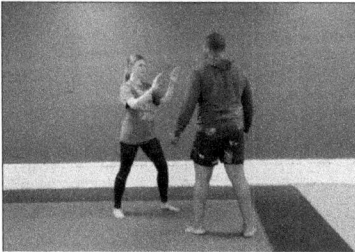

Intuition is probably the most overlooked capability you have available. It can assist you in avoiding away from danger. Similar to Spider-Man's spider-sense , which makes him able to detect danger before it is too late, intuition works in a similar way. Intuition refers to the feeling that you have inside your gut that, despite whatever evidence you have it is telling that you should avoid a certain location, person or even a the situation.

We all know that guys tend to be a bit snobby. We've long since lost all connection to our basic intuition. You'll not find many YouTube videos of women smoking bottle rockets with their mouths on the 4th of July. However, there are many more I'm happy to have counted of guys who have done it. Fire and mouth aren't a good combination. Men who had strong ability to sense intuition(and basic sense) this would not be the case. Women have an enthralling connection with their own inner voice.

As you are getting in an Uber You notice something appears suspicious regarding the driver. You decide not to continue climbing into the car to avoid being uncomfortable. You inform them that they can go on without you. You need to complete some work.

Personal Note: This incident is very personal to me as it was the case for my wife, who had a drink with a bunch of friends. After an evening of food as well as drinks requested an Uber for the group to take home. As they drove they could tell that his mood was not right. In no time, they jumped out as quickly as that was available and instructed the driver to not take the fare and to keep going.

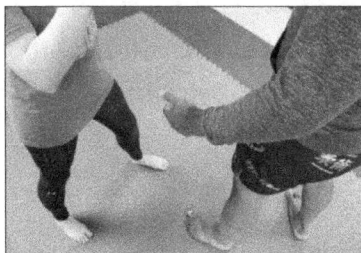

*You finally are invited to a dinner party with a brand new group, but there's a catch. Your friends can't be there with you. You're determined to increase your circle of friends, you aren't worried about it as you'll take a few drinks and leave the party early. Just a few minutes away from leaving the party, a person keeps coming up to you and offer you an alcohol drink even though you've declined. He insists that you relax, but your intuition tells you that isn't the case. There's something you don't like with him and his drink. Leave because your instinct will not let you go.

While it could appear to be mystical and mysterious, intuition isn't. Scientists believe that intuition is in the ability to gather sensory information in hundreds of seconds that creates a picture of an event or even a person. It's a combination of how someone stands or smiles, speaks and moves, dress or how a space might smell or look.

It is our evolution from Jiminy Cricket. We hear it chirping in our ears, leading us to security.

Don't be afraid to trust your instincts. It's not a fading quality as an appendix. If your choice is to listen to the voice of your heart, or taking a risk in a scenario that you're not sure about, listen to the wisdom of Jiminy, rely on your gut instinct and be cautiously.

I would be utterly indecent if I did not take this opportunity to highlight Gavin de Beckers' book The Gift Of Fear. Gavin's Gift of Fear is a excellently written exploration of the nature of intuition as well as its connection to fears and the need to survive. There are many stories in the book that are not just relevant, but each could transform your life. This is the book that I would recommend for each self-defense class I teach.

Even monkeys get thrown out of trees. This is why we all make mistakes, even though we're skilled in our job. Even with the best efforts made using situationsal awareness, intuition mental modeling, and other tools available to us If you are in the presence of an adversary in the area, de-escalation is the next step to take.

De-escalation as well as the Interview

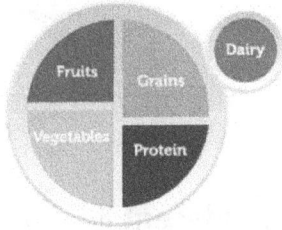

The interview stance and de-escalation are inextricably related. De-escalation can be described as the ability to decrease or completely fall off an opponent's defense so that we can be able to escape or take action first. The response of our attempts to deescalate, will determine the direction of our actions rather than the reverse. But avoiding conflicts with physical force is the the top prioritization.

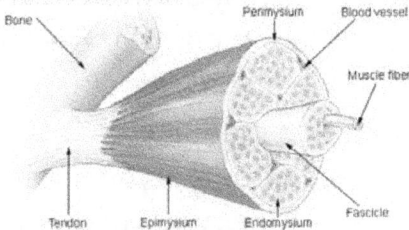

(A1)Eva's pose and posture are not hostile. When she holds her hands she is able to be offensive or defensive at a moment's notice.

(A2)Notice Eva's hips and feet are situated off of my center. This gives her the power to be directed to me.

Like the image above(A1) In the above image (A1), the interview stance is one that, in its own way, seems to be non-confrontational however, it places you in a the position of launching or defending an attack as quickly as possible while limiting the distance between yourself and the attacker. This tactic is frequently employed by law enforcement personnel when communicating with individuals on an emergency call. The protector is placed in the middle of the person who is likely to be the aggressor, at roughly 45 degrees angle. The guard's hands are raised with their index fingers and thumbs framing their face like they are in an image frame.

Beware that the risk is conducting an interview with you simultaneously. They are monitoring your responses to their questions, or their presence to determine if you're an apex threat. The first few seconds are crucial for this.

The first and most important thing is that any attempts to deescalate must be made from our interview position. If you have your hands down and you're standing directly in front of the threat and are not able to move, we're more vulnerable to being seen as prey and being snatched away.

There are two approaches to de-escalation. I prefer to consider them as hard or soft strategies. They are not the ultimate method. The mindset of the opponent and their tactics determine the best strategy of de-escalation we choose to use.

The gentle method of de-escalation is a more flexible approach that allows the player to play alongside the attacker. You do not stare them directly in their eye and you don't keep a good posture. Perhaps you stumble over your words. You could call it submissive or kowtowing and yet there's an advantage to this approach. The more confident your adversary is and the more confident they are, the less likely they perceive you as an enemy. Consider it as verbal jiu-Jitsu.

Example A:

Affliction:" Why are you acting like a jerk, I just wanted not to offend you!"

Protectionist: "I'm sorry, it is a really difficult week. My dog passed away recently and has been making me tear up all week."

In this instance, I didn't provide a solution which allowed them to increase the agression. I didn't provide them with anything that would contradict their views. In fact, I sided with the views of them. It's about trying to guide them in a way that doesn't conflict with them. Imagine it as a sales task. The more you debate with your customer even if your argument is rational more likely you are to win the deal. In this case what you're selling is your security.

The soft method can make the person who is observing you incredibly dangerous as they aren't aware of your real motives or the devastating destruction you could do to them, should you need to. Since you're under control, or simply plosoftg along to give you to put yourself in a safe area or near weapons that are environmentally friendly, such as the lamp or pen. When you are taking a gentle approach, it's crucial to establish an overall strategy. If you're waiting on the situation to change and slow down, don't wait to grab the opportunity to escape when an opportunity arises.

The hard method is an even more direct and hard-nosed approach to dealing the aggressor. In the moment of confrontation The hard approach deal with the aggressor's questions by taking them to the eye while remaining confident and not retreating. The objective is to show an assertive front and warn the offender that getting you into trouble could result in a life-altering event for them.

There is a good chance that you've encountered people you encounter at work, school or at the gym and you think to yourself "that person seems very serious I would not want to play with them." This attitude isn't the best one to adopt. You need to feel confident in yourself to convey that confidence in the first few seconds of your interview. The disadvantage of the method that is hard is that the more confident you are during the conversation the more likely people are to be more vigilant and make it more difficult to control the situation.

Which defense method is more effective either hard or soft? It depends. It is dependent on your personal situation, your surroundings and most importantly, it is dependent on your risk. That's why being aware of your own intuition will be vital. It is possible to start with a strict approach, and change to a more gentle approach once the situation has changed.

Steps to Action

How can you practice de-escalation

A technique I employ is to include one person whose sole purpose is to stop a conflict against the aggressor. We usually start without striking, however this may change in later phases when we introduce more issues. The person who is the aggressor (Partner B) may be a drunk man in a bar, or a driver who is prone to road anger. Whatever the situation you are dealing with, it must fit into your life. If you do not frequent bars, there's no sense to play out scenarios in the bar. In general, the partner B will have a predetermined reaction to either de-escalate or attack and only according to the actions of the protector. The better the performance of partner A in de-escalating, the more likely that Partner B will be able to de-escalate too.

A protector (Partner A) attempts to calm the person until they calm them down or go out on their own. When you practice soft or hard make sure you speak in a clear and even tone. Be aware of your words before speaking. It's all about how you act. You either appear confident or you appear like you don't have confidence. You sell it by how you move. If you've had experience in theatre in improvisation, then you'll enjoy this exercise.

Although this is only an exercise, anyone who approaches your as an aggressor real life typically isn't in a rational state of mind, that trying to use logic alone to find your way out might not be the most effective strategy. The more you work on your feet , and mastering the ability to stay clear of the traps that follow and the more confident you will be in your self-defense capabilities.

The most common mistakes to avoid when trying de-escalation

*Please Please, please, don't advise the other person to, "calm down". This hasn't been successful throughout the history of humanity. It's going to produce the opposite impact.

Do not belittle them in front acquaintances. If their self-esteem is damaged then their guards are raised , and they are more risky.

Don't be threatening with them. This can trigger an involuntary response from them to raise their security..

*Don't let them know you're prepared to fight. It's an instant rise for them. This is the same as telling the police that you're planning to rob a bank because you're on the route toward the banks.

The best result in this scenario is that a punch or kick does not occur and you can go home safe. In spite of all your efforts, you are not able to convince the person to resign, regardless of whether it's your partner or a complete stranger and you're faced with only one option. Make the effort to escape safely and then act immediately.

Preemption

If everything else fails and it appears that violence is imminent, you have the possibility of defending yourself when you think your safety is in danger. It is common knowledge it is the person who first to strike punches is the one who gets into trouble with the law. It's not the way it operates.

In the context of the United States (check your local laws, I'm not an attorney) Physical contact is not required for an incident to be deemed an assault. An assault could include a threat to speak with which I declare my intention clear that I will do you bodily harm , and I'm totally capable of doing this. If I phone you via phone and say I'm going to "fight you" and I'm located in North Carolina and you are located in California It could be unlawful for me to verbally threaten you however there isn't a chance of bodily harm because of the distance. So, you cannot fly in North Carolina and fight me since I threatened you on the phone.

If, however, we're crossing each other's street and come across one another Then, with my face smacked with a scowl, I tell you, "I'm going to beat your back." Have I communicate my intention clearly? Are I equipped with the tools to accomplish this? If you think your safety is in danger you are entitled to safeguard yourself by hitting first when retreat is not feasible.

It is important to be aware of the laws here , but we do not want to confuse the waters excessively, for two reasons. The first is that you must be aware of self-defense laws that apply to the location you live in. There are two books written exclusively on self-defense and the law. They are searchable on the internet. However, for many fighting for their rights is difficult enough without worrying about the consequences to come.

This is the time to exercise the common sense. We shouldn't hit people simply because they saw us in the wrong way or took our parking space out. It is important to be real-to-life anxiety that should we not take action now we may never have an opportunity to do so again. When we engage with the danger, it is important to can only can stop the threat for so that we can escape. If we do manage to get them down then don't kick them for the reason that they are not worthy of it(unless they're still attacking you). The most important thing about self-defense is that it does not be a punishment.

When I use neutralizing threats, exactly what does it mean? Simply, if it is needed we fight hard and long enough to ensure that the threat:

1.Unable or unwilling engage in combat.

2.Is shocked, disoriented or hurt for enough to quit the scene.

Why is it important to be first? Because it's superior to being last. If we're not the first, in this case we're the last. Whoever is first puts the other to enter an emotional state. What is more effective reacting or taking action? In this instance, action is. If you are waiting for them to grab or hit your body, you're already in the back of. In general, the person who is first, in any self-defense incident is the one who gets and holds the advantage. We're after an upper hand and not their.

If this is a good fit for you, or isn't send a message to social media using the #BeFirst as well as the #SimplySelfDefense hashtags. Let me know your thoughts I'd like to hear from you.

Chapter 19: Understanding The Human Body

In this section we'll explore how the body works and the way it functions. This information is essential to be aware of what you should do and not do to maximize your workout sessions. This information will assist you in getting results faster especially when you're striving to improve your physical strength. In the beginning, we'll discuss nutrition and how your body makes use of energy. After that, we'll discuss the skeletal muscles.

Nutrition The way our bodies function

The first thing we need to do is be aware of where our body's energy originates. This is crucial because we have to understand the best sources of energy that we can select. Grappling is an activity that demands a lot energy. To be a good grappler, you need to be able to replenish with energy and strengthen your body.

Every living thing requires an element of nutrition in order they be able to utilize energy for any need. Plants require nutrients from the soil and also energy from sunlight. Human beings, as well as many other animals as well, get their nutrients by eating food. The measurement of energy is via the Calorie (also called 1000 calories or a Kilocalorie). Calorie is a measure of energy. Calorie is a measurement of heat that is a type of energy. Your body store calories that are digested from foods and uses them as needed. In layman's terms, one could say that the reason we feel our temperature rises when we exercise is due to the fact of the body's release of energy stored in the calories. In the average, humans should consume between 1800-2000 Calories each day. The nutritional requirements prohibit consuming less than 1500 calories so that the body is able to perform its functions normal.

There are three main groups that you must keep in mind when discussing nutrition. These are macronutrients and minerals, and vitamins. The two latter are vital to maintain good health, however, they are not always associated in energy. We will therefore begin by discussing macronutrients.

The body requires this first group of nutrients in huge quantities. This is due to the fact that the body converts the macronutrients category into energy. In the absence of energy, your body is starving and it will greatly hinder your everyday functioning. The three main components of macronutrients include carbohydrates, fats and proteins. These two are the major sources of energy.

Carbohydrates constitute a significant proportion in our daily diets. They are present in nearly every food item, but they are more prevalent in fruits. Examples of carbohydrates include sugars along with fibers and starches. Pasta, candies, and any other sweet or starchy food items are rich in carbohydrates. Once metabolized, carbohydrates create about 4 Calories per grams.

The fats in meat are much more plentiful meat than in plants. The most common examples of fats are oils, lard and the fat that is attached to meat. The body generally burns carbohydrates first , then fat. This is why more people are overweight. The fats that they are taking is not burning off, but are instead stored. This is unnatural since fats emit greater Calories in a gram than carbohydrates. However, it's better for weight loss to cut down on consumption of carbs rather than fats.

Some fats aren't beneficial. In excess consumption of trans and saturated fats (which you can monitor by looking at the nutritional information found on the label of the product) can increase the Low Density Lipoprotein (LDL) levels of cholesterol and lower HDL levels. Lipoprotein (HDL) the levels of cholesterol. LDL is often referred to as the"bad cholesterol". The increased consumption of LDLs could cause obstructions in blood vessels, resulting in an increase in blood pressure and the chance of suffering from heart attacks.

Once metabolized, fats offer about 9 Calories per Gram.

Proteins are also plentiful in meats, as well as certain varieties of plants. They help to create, maintain, and repair muscles, as well as different kinds of cells. Because of these characteristics that the body uses up proteins to generate energy for the duration of. Maintaining a high protein diet can help burn fat. In general, if you're trying to build muscle, you should consume 1gram of protein for every pounds of body mass. As they are metabolized, proteins offer approximately 4 Calories per Gram.

Minerals and vitamins are instances of micronutrients. Contrary to macronutrients you only require them in tiny amounts. In reality, excessive consumption of certain kinds of micronutrients may cause severe health issues. But the majority of diets are already enriched with micronutrients that they are not deficient. The problem is when you eat the same food every day.

In general it's a good idea to adhere to the MyPlate plan to know the amount of a particular food item to consume. MyPlate is the food guide offered to the United States Department of Agriculture to ensure that people receive the right amount of nutrients. It was created to replace Food Pyramid. Food Pyramid which put a major emphasis on starchy carbohydrates foods like pasta and bread.

The MyPlate system ensures you don't suffer from any nutritional deficiency. Image is taken directly from United States Department of Agriculture (n.d.).

The idea behind MyPlate is to split portions of your meal into 4 distinct wedges sizes , and to you can also add a glass or small dish of dairy. The largest wedge of your plate is the quantity of vegetables you must consume. Vegetables have low calories however, they are full of macronutrients as well as micronutrients. Grains are the second most significant portion. They supply you with carbohydrates to ensure that you get the energy you require for the entire day. A third of the wedge contains proteins to help you construct as well as repair cells. The tiniest wedge on the plate is made for fruits. Fruits are rich in sugar, yet they are rich in micronutrients, and it is essential to consume only a tiny amount of fruit in your daily diet. In addition, dairy helps to address the absence of fat on the plate and will also provide micronutrients that might not have been gotten from the wedges on the plate.

A balanced intake of macronutrients and micronutrients is essential to maintain a proper nutrition balance. The final thing to consider is water. If you are active and sweat, you will sweat. Drinking water is essential to stay hydrated. But, electrolytes and minerals can also be ejected from your body via sweat. So, it's better to drink diluted fruit juices to replenish the micronutrients that have been lost. Concentrated juices contain excessive sugar, and should not be recommended for exercise.

How can we move forward?

Bones play a role in keeping us in a straight and mobile position. Every bone plays a role in the sense of contributing to body shape, balance or strength. Grappling calls for specific muscles, known as muscles of the skeletal system to perform the required movements and gestures.

To show how muscles function Imagine that your muscles consist of strings that are thin and are able to slide across each other when employed. These strings are known as muscle fibers and make the muscles tight and relax in order to facilitate movements. In general, muscles are required to relax or contract during any one movement. If that weren't the case, then movement could be static and mechanical even if you were able to move even. It is recommended to build your muscles in order that you are able to execute proper grappling technique and moves without overstretching your skeletal muscles or causing injuries.

The skeletal muscle is connected to bone via muscles and is comprised of many strings known as muscle fibers. (Darling, n.d.)

The two kinds of skeletal muscles are red muscle, which is slow and the faster or white muscle. The slow muscle is made up of Type 1 muscles that enable the muscle to withstand strain. This muscle is essential in grappling since you'd like to stay in a straight line and be anchored to the ground, without your muscles weak. The fast muscle makes use of Type two muscle fibers which permit quick bursts of movement. This kind of muscle isn't as crucial in grappling as agility is not often required in comparison to endurance and brute strength. But, they do fatigue faster than slower muscles and must still be developed to last longer during training.

Every person has a unique proportion of the two kinds. There are some who are extremely quick and can be able to endure extended periods of running and jumping. There are also individuals can endure prolonged durations of walking or climbing. It is a result of genetics, however it can be altered. If you do not possess a specific type of fibers in your muscles, it is possible to exercise them through continuous tasks that require the muscles.

In order to become a proficient grappler, you need to be able to build the type 1 muscles in order to grow your red muscle. This will enable you to become more durable as Milo of Croton and having the same strength as his. To strengthen to build your Type 1 , muscle fibers you need to do a lot of exercises for strength. This will be covered in the following chapter. It may be beneficial to have the correct muscle ratio, but don't be discouraged if you're genetically handicapped. All you have to keep in mind when you are a beginner is to train yourself into an effective and proficient grappler.

Chapter 20: Self-Defense for Teens - What is the Best?

I get asked frequently what the impact of using force is on different standards for juveniles.

Recently, a student at one of our classes shared his daughter, who was 16 years old, was assaulted by a more mature female right after she left their school bus. It was a gorgeous day with no sign of danger. After the school bus had left at this particular location his daughter was snatched from behind by her hair and dragged to the floor. The female attacker jumped over her, then slammed her head against the ground and then proceeded to smash her nose.

The daughter's companion tried to get the attacker away from her, but this was impeded by two men who were watching the show. They probably were with the attacker and dragged the girl's friend off without allowing her to interfere further. In the vicinity, a few others were watching and doing nothing. Some of them were cheering for the attacker. One witness phoned the police and obtained the license number of the vehicle which left the scene along with the attacker and her male companions.

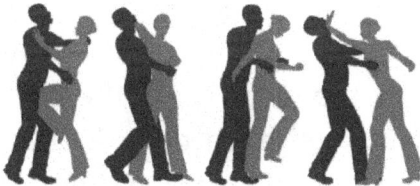

The person who takes part in our class reacted as every other father concerned His daughter was brutally attacked, for no reason. The father's anger was quite understandable. Following the incident, the police probed the incident and found the perpetrator and her accomplices. The suspect, who was an older adult who was in probation. The case will be pounded throughout the justice system, and we can only hope that the outcome will please the victim and her parents.

In the aftermath of this attack, the father asked me how my daughter could have protected herself. The answer is that she has the same right to self-defense just like any other civilian within the state. In Minnesota one can be aged 16 years old or older "may have and utilize an approved tear gas mixture in the exercise of reasonable force for defense of the individual or the property of the person in the event it is released out of an aerosol container that is marked with clear instructions on the use of the product, and is date-stamped to show its expected use." An individual who is 18 years old or more experienced "may have and utilize an electronic incantation device for the use of reasonable force for defense of the individual or the property of the individual only when the electronic device is marked with the appropriate clearly written instructions regarding its usage and the risks associated in its use." Then, lastly: "Reasonable force may be applied to or against the person of another , without consent from the other party if the conditions are in place or the user reasonably believes they exist ....When employed by anyone who is resistance or in aiding another person to resist an attack against another."

From the legal standpoint she was entitled to the right to use reasonable force in order to protect her. It would have been appropriate for her to have employed tear gas or pepper spray, or an electronic device for incantation against an attacker who was attempting to crush her head against the ground.

The father's question presents an interesting problem. Minnesota state laws don't permit firearms within the school premises. It is against the law of the state for a girl to possess any firearm while at school. The girl is in a school that has an zero tolerance policy for any type of weapon. The young lady had just completed her school day and got on a bus that was provided by her school. The school district is liable for some accountability to ensure the safety of the young lady during her time at school, and up to the point that she leaves the bus. Once she steps off the bus, she's alone with no one else. Now what?

The 16-year-old student can carry mace pepper spray or tear gas compound when she gets off the bus. What, if anything, can she get it if she's been spending the entire day in situations where it's either unlawful or in violation of an rules to have something like this?

The majority of states in the Assembled States have enacted similar laws to the one taken from Minnesota: "whoever possesses, keeps, or stores any dangerous weapon or makes use of or displays an imitation firearm or firearm that is a BB while being in school premises is guilty of a criminal offense and may be punished by jail for not more than two years, or to the payment of a fine less than $5,000, and/or both." Schools have policies that are based on the laws. A number of decades of shooters (counting school shootings) and gang violence has produced these policies and laws that are geared towards preventing violence and limiting the liability. But this is the reason they've caused yet another problem.

Apart from the laws mentioned above, many states have legislation that are similar to Minnesota's law in the area of self-defense. "Reasonable force can be used against or in the direction of another person without their consent if the circumstances exist or the user reasonably believes that they do exist. ....When employed by anyone who is resistance or in aiding someone else in resisting an offense against another ......When employed by an individual who is in lawful possession of personal or tangible assets, as well as by a person helping the person who is who is in lawful possession of the property, to resist a trespass on or other illegal obstruction to the property ..."

In other words, you may use reasonable force against someone without their consent in the event you believe they're trying to harm yourself or another person or you are able to trust them to not attempt to take your property or the property of someone else. This man's 16 year old daughter. The circumstance she encountered on that day, and the current laws in force, leaves her with no option to protect herself other than with hands. Anything she can use her hands to do that could be considered "reasonable" in the eyes of the law are her only alternatives.

The woman suffered the injury of a fractured nose, which required some surgical intervention. Restitution is a possibility in court, it's much more often unpredictable than it is gathered successfully. We should move this situation an additional step. What happens if she kicked the bucket because of her head being struck on the concrete floor? Does anyone have a responsibility on their side? I'm not able to provide an answer to thatquestion, however we could throw in some additional hypothetical elements to give it some interest.

The young lady had made a complaint to school officials about being frequently being scolded by a woman at the bus stop. Her father approached school officials asking the permission of his child to wear pepper spray as a result due to the severity of violence. School officials declined the request. In the present, what kind of legal case can be made to prove responsibility? Negligence is defined by a person's inability to exercise the judgment and diligence that a sensible person would use in similar circumstances in order to avoid the possibility of harm to another.

In a civil case usually, the plaintiff will be given restitution, compensation or compensation for their loss:

* The defendant was under the duty of care;

* The defendant was unable to meet this obligation;

* This negligence led to the plaintiff's injury or death;

* The actual damage resulted from the damages.

The term "gross negligence" is generally defined as an act or omission that is committed in reckless disregard for the consequences that affect someone's life or assets of an individual. That leaves us with many questions to think about. Should schools offer self-defense classes in their regular curriculum? Should parents assume the responsibility of selecting their children for self-defense classes? Are state laws and government school system policies been too far in trying to protect students and reduce the violence?

These laws and regulations are put in place with an underlying reason. In all likelihood when they are in a situation like this one, they can also be the self-defense options. Similar to this there are schools that have zero-brutality policy. I remember a time when my son intervened the event that one of his classmates was being assaulted in the school. My son intervened and pushed the attacker away from his partner and then threw the attacker to the floor. My son was placed in immobilization in the school for several days, as was his friend and the attacker. The school did not care about officials, who took whatever action during the incident. They took an approach of shotgun to these issues; everyone is liable.

I had a great conversation about his counselor, and his guidance counselor about the "bad habit" rule in the school a few days afterward. I went over the statutes concerning reasonable force and told them that they have no legal right to take these rights from students. They agreed that this was likely correct and said they would get legal counsel to investigate the matter. This is a new dilemma. The school arrangement appears to override the laws of the state. In general, any private or open element like a school corporate, or other organisation can limit significantly more in the manner of approaching the laws allow. For instance, despite possibility that I'm an valid gun permit holder, as is permitted by law in the state my boss can prohibit guns from their premises. It's fine. But, as it happens in the case of the use of reasonable force to protect you or others, some schools are in a risky situation since there is law of the land which outlines the right to protect yourself regardless of the location you are.

Primarily Consideration

There is no substance that could take this fundamental principle to defend yourself. This doesn't mean that people who practice it will not be held accountable for their actions as so, but you must be ready to protect your actions from the legal standpoint.

Chapter 21: What Should You Do If You've Got Multiple Attackers?

With several attackers, it could be the most stressful, chaotic and frightening situations you'll ever encounter, so it's best to prepare. There are a lot of punches, and defenses will not work in this situation since when you fight or punch to one opponent, the other is likely to come at you. Strategies and tactics are the most important elements in this scenario. We have listed below some strategies and techniques which will definitely help in the event that you find yourself in a situation.

Continuously Unpredictable Movements

Change your position constantly Moving targets are difficult to smash. Perform different moves and attacks It will be hard for attackers to create a trap against you. This could create confusion among them, and also result in your attackers falling and hitting themselves.

175

Shielding

It is impossible to tackle each attacker at the at the same time. A strategy to be able to take on them one at a time is known as shielding. The first step is choosing an attacker, and drawing him closer to you. Then, you can make him a shield against other attackers who appear to be more formidable. This means that you will use one attacker to protect yourself against more powerful attackers.

Redirection and Deflection

The attackers in groups never organize their attacks They aren't trained and, of course, their strength lies in their numbers , so they do not bother with training or any of that. When taking that into consideration, a smart strategy is to deflect and redirect members toward one another or towards surrounding environment, like barriers, fences or vehicles. Deflecting requires sidestepping, dithering pulling and shoving. these actions ensure that they are not off balance. In addition, redirection requires pushing, shoving and pulling of the attackers towards each other or to other objects.

The Busting Out

This technique is very useful in situations when you discover yourself in a tight spot. You search for a gap between the group members, and then you push yourself to run and break free into the space to get out of. If there's no space, search for a person you consider to be"the weak link "weak link" and then smash this person. You could attack him or be loud enough to push rid of him.

Use Your Environment

Concentrate on locations in your environment which can give you an advantage. If you notice areas that are geared towards them, it can lower the chance that the attacker will strike. Choose a location that is well lit even if you're in a dark location as you'll be able to spot their actions and the chance of others observing you in the middle of a crisis will be greater. Install some barriers, such as vehicles in between you and your adversaries. Keep in mind potential weapons to use such as bottles, bats, boards, etc.

Get away in the Right Time

Escape from an attack group appears to be the most logical and rational decision to make. The issue is, what if they had weapons? When you turn and run, you'll be subject to shots from guns. If the worst-case scenario occurs, you'll be exhausted and your ability to fight diminished and it may not be a good moment to escape.

Be Safe for Your Family and Friends

Being a victim of a gang can be a nightmare and having someone you love with you when it happens can make things more complicated. You cannot just flee and go away. Neither do you want to attack them without thinking or attack the person you are attacking. If an attacker is able to get hold of your loved one , they will surely gain the psychological and strategic advantage. The only way to deal with this scenario is to prevent them from gaining access to your loved one at all costs.

Priority Goals

It's not enough just to are able to punch but you also need to learn how to use your punches. A single punch could have numerous effects based on the area of the body it hits. For example, a strike on the arm won't cause more than a blow to the eye. Make sure you target those four Ns to prevent rapid and painful injuries including neck, Nose, Nuts and knees.

Chapter 22: Top Pressure Point Targets for Beginners

In this article, we'll explore some of the top pressure points on the body that you must take on to protect yourself effectively. It is important to note that these are the same points that are used in both the acupressure and acupuncture. Certain of these points are often pressurized or massaged to aid in healing.

The pressure points mentioned in this chapter are specifically chosen for complete beginners. It is not necessary to know how to perform advanced forms of kicks or punches to get those pressure points.

But, it is important to remember that hitting them with force will create a number of negative effects on your body. The majority of the time the pressure points result in severe discomfort. The pressure points that are hit will cause knees to flex. In the next chapter, we'll explain how to target specific pressure points to take out the attacker.

Pressure Point: Lung 8

Lung 8 is also referred to for its radial nerve. It is an excellent area of attack since it can be used for numerous practical applications in the streets. Additionally it's popular with novices who are still learning the basics of pressure point combat and self-defense.

It's actually one those pressure points on your body that you will not be scared to hit because it's on the arm, which is why you would think that it won't be a direct influence on the whole body.

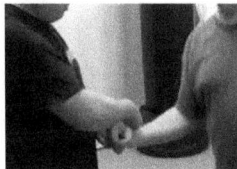

The term "lung 8" is used to describe Lung 8 since it triggers an action reflex to the lung. In the traditional Chinese medicine the pressure point is located on what is known as "the lung line in the body" (an entire nerve line that influence the lung).

Be aware that the pressure point is mostly an area of rub which means that you rub the spot to trigger a reaction from the body. But that isn't a guarantee that you'll rub it while fighting with someone.

It is possible to punch it. You can also grasp it and press it against the aforementioned point with the force and power of your hands.

This is a hint: when you hit the lung #8, you must to hit it with 45 degrees (or similar to it) and your rub or strike should be directed towards the hand, not towards the elbow.

Where can I find it?

This is where you'll locate that pressure spot:

If you look in the above picture there are already two lung points located along the forearm's ridge (the one on the thumb). It is not necessary to be extremely precise when trying to hit this point as it's easy to find and hit.

To locate the pressure point correctly in training and practice Find the inside of your wrist. Three finger widths are measured from the line or crease. The point will be on the indentation of two bones that connect towards the wrist, which are called the radial bone. It is known as the Lung Eight point situated in the bone of the radial on the thumb's side. It is shaped like an Y-shaped letter.

Conclusion

The topics discussed here are only a brief overview of the laws that govern the use the use of deadly force in self-defense. The laws are continuously being revised and changed. In addition, case and court decisions tend to be different every time, since the rulings depend on the way in which the event happened as well as how jurors and judges consider the situation.

The principles that are presented here are designed to provide you with an understanding of when it could be absolute necessity to use deadly force. However, there are certain circumstances that could justify the need to use deadly force, however it doesn't protect the individual from civil liability. One of the best ways to ensure that you are secure is to exercise restraint and alertness throughout the day.